A Guide to
ALZHEIMER'S
DISEASE

A Guide to ALZHEIMER'S DISEASE

Barry Reisberg, M.D.

THE FREE PRESS
A Division of Macmillan, Inc.
NEW YORK

Collier Macmillan Publishers
LONDON

The Free Press
A Division of Macmillan, Inc.
866 Third Avenue, New York, N. Y. 10022

Collier Macmillan Canada, Inc.

First Free Press Paperback Edition 1983

Printed in the United States of America

printing number

      7 8 9 10

Library of Congress Cataloging in Publication Data

Reisberg, Barry.
   A guide to Alzheimer's disease.

   Rev. ed. of: Brain failure. c1981.
   Bibliography: p.
   Includes index.
   1. Alzheimer's disease. I. Reisberg, Barry. Brain
failure. II. Title.
RC523.R44 1983   616.89 '83   83-20511
  ISBN 0-02-926370-0 (pbk.)
This book was previously published in hardbound edition under the title BRAIN FAILURE,
An Introduction to Current Concepts of Senility, 1981.

*Dedicated in Memory
of Rosalie*

"Truth . . . is a great coquette, she will not be sought with too much passion, but often is most amenable to indifference. She escapes when apparently caught, but gives herself up if patiently waited for; revealing herself after farewells have been said, but inexorable when loved with too much fervor."

Ernest Renan, speech welcoming
Louis Pasteur to the Académie Française, 1882

Contents

Contents

Foreword
by Robert N. Butler, M.D.

AGING HAS LONG BEEN MISTAKENLY EQUATED with disease and an inevitable downhill pattern in both physical and mental functioning. Nowhere is this more evident than in the treatment—or rather lack of treatment—of mental impairment in the elderly.

It is currently estimated that between 500,000 and 1.5 million persons suffer from the more serious and irreversible forms of senile dementia. Approximately 50 percent of all nursing home residents have some degree of mental impairment, with Alzheimer's disease being a major reason for admissions to nursing homes. Given that few trends are as evident or predictable as the aging of the American population, those responsible for scientific research and service delivery are facing a series of challenges. A key element in our preparation for the future and for large numbers of persons surviving into old age must be research aimed at increasing our knowledge of the causes and the biological and behavioral mechanisms at work in senile dementia. Such research would improve our ability to treat and control these devastating conditions which take their toll primarily in the elderly population, and perhaps eventually to prevent these diseases altogether.

The insidious onset and progressive development of conditions such as senile dementia demand that we study disease in old age as a developmental process and not merely as an isolated acute event. In research this calls for multidisciplinary studies such as those supported under the broad mandate of the National Institute on Aging. The legislation which established the NIA called for the "conduct and support of biomedical, social, and behavioral research and training related to the aging process and the diseases and other special problems and needs of the aged."

Since the creation of the NIA in 1974, there have been a number of efforts throughout the federal government to sponsor research on senile dementia. Most recently, the Institute coordinated a health research initiative on Alzheimer's disease and the dementias of aging. This initiative represents the individual and cooperative activities of the NIA, the National Institute of Neurological and Communicative Disorders and Stroke, the National Institute of Mental Health, the National Institute of Allergy and Infectious Diseases, and the National Institute for Occupational Safety and Health.

The changing demographic profile of the American population also requires that we properly train students in all areas of the health professions to provide sensitive care and effective treatment for the patients they will be serving. Fortunately, health care professionals are beginning to respond to the realities of practice by demanding information on the special needs and problems of elderly patients. Through mechanisms like the NIA Geriatric Medicine Academic Award, a number of medical schools are incorporating geriatrics into their curricula and practical training experiences. Still, physicians, and particularly psychiatrists, too often fail to see the older person as a candidate for successful treatment. There need to be major reforms in all medical schools, with the strong support of departments of psychiatry. We need to introduce and to require human development courses which cover all stages of life from birth until death, and to develop psychiatric residency programs which include experiences with older patients in all major diagnostic categories.

With regard to treatment, the chronic and complex nature of senile dementia requires that we make use of the best available knowledge in the fields of internal medicine, neurology, psychiatry, epidemiology, radiology, psychology, geriatric medicine, general medicine, and pharmacology. More sensitive and reliable techniques are needed for the diagnosis of Alzheimer's disease and to identify persons with treatable forms of mental impairment. In particular, there is a need for the development of more sophisticated psychological tests to parallel the remarkable advances in our ability to depict the structure and function of the brain in a noninvasive manner.

In *A Guide to Alzheimer's Disease,* Dr. Reisberg ably describes the historical developments which have revolutionized our thinking with regard to mental impairment in old age, as well as current methods for diagnosis and treatment. He also reviews the fast-breaking and exciting research advances in the fields of neuropathology, biochemistry, endocrinology, immunology, virology, toxicology, and genetics, which are opening the way to an understanding of the causes and mechanisms of Alzheimer's disease. It may be that no one of the current research leads will give us the means to prevent Alzheimer's disease. But at the very least, the growing interest in research on the dementias of age gives hope that an effective treatment will eventually be found.

Acknowledgments

THIS WORK WOULD NOT HAVE BEEN POSSIBLE without the continuing stimulation and ongoing support I have received from many sources. Some of these sources are particularly noteworthy.

Samuel Gershon, M.D., placed me in a position in which I was permitted the luxury of studying and observing geriatric patients. Sam's warmth and wisdom nourished me continually during my early experiences in geriatric psychiatry.

Steven H. Ferris, Ph.D., shared his knowledge, insights, and astute observations from his experience in research with memory problems in geriatric patients. Steve has remained an invaluable associate, companion, and intellectual resource.

Several of my other associates at the Neuropsychopharmacology Research Unit and at the Geriatric Study Program provided the creative and intellectual milieu that fosters original investigation. One of those worthy of particular note is Mony J. de Leon, Ed.D., a companion and fellow explorer of, until recently, a neglected field. Others who have followed parallel but occasionally intersecting paths have included John Rotrosen, M.D.; Burton Angrist, M.D.; Michael Stanley, Ph.D.; Eitan Friedman, Ph.D.; Anastase Georgotas, M.D.; and John Mann, M.D.

Introducing junior associates to a new and growing discipline can be as rewarding an experience as any. For this privilege, I would like to thank my research psychiatric fellows Michael Schneck, M.D., and Nunzio Pomara, M.D.

Robert Cancro, M.D., has been a noteworthy source of continual support without whose assistance my own investigations and those of all the scientists whom I have named above would not have been possible.

My own investigations have also been assisted by funds from the National Institute of Aging, the National Institute of Mental Health, and the National Institute of Neurological, Communicative Disease and Stroke.

A source of knowledge and of comfort as important as any of the above-named persons has been the patients of the Geriatric Study and Treatment Program of the Department of Psychiatry at N.Y.U. Our patients as a group are to be commended for their cooperation and their willingness to serve as the wellsprings from which further knowledge of the field must flow. The information contained in this volume is ample testimony to the insights they have provided.

On a more personal level, I would like to take this opportunity to thank my mother, Claire, for her patience and interest in listening to every word of this document, so as to ensure its complete comprehensibility to laymen as well as to professionals. I would also like to thank Turan Itil, M.D., for his crucial assistance in introducing me to the world of psychiatric research, a world that I find inestimably exciting and extraordinarily promising.

                                                                    B.R.

Chapter 1

The Rediscovery of Senile Brain Failure

BRAIN FAILURE, LIKE OLD AGE, is a condition which mankind has always reluctantly recognized and always accepted—with resignation. So closely have people associated the loss of intellectual functioning with normal aging that they have not always found it necessary to have different words for the two conditions. Indeed one word is currently used to refer to the two states of aging and loss of intellect: "senility." The 1975 unabridged second edition of *Webster's New Twentieth Century Dictionary* defines senility as:

"old age"
"weakness"
"the characteristics of old age"
"infirmity of mind and body"[1]

Old age is certainly not synonymous with loss of intellectual functioning. Indeed, we now know that many people enter their seventh, eighth, and ninth decades with no measurable decline in their intellectual functioning from that in their youth or their middle age.[2] Conversely, some persons undergo intellectual decline in their fifth or sixth decade. When this early intellectual decline does occur, it is not accompanied by the other changes which all of us associate with aging. The skin retains the firmness and resilience of middle age. Arthritis, with its characteristic effects on posture and on facility of movement, is no more likely to occur. Nor are the sensory changes which we know to be increasingly frequent as people age more likely to become manifest at an earlier age if brain failure occurs unusually early in life. Persons with early onset of brain failure, or "presenile dementia," as it is called, are no more likely to develop cataracts or loss of auditory acuity than other persons their own age. Indeed, changes in many bodily functions are more closely related to chronological aging than the intellectual changes which we associate with being senile.[3]

In one sense the intellectual decline, or "dementia," which we associate with senility is related to old age. The incidence of the intellectual deterioration does appear to increase steadily with age from the fifth decade to the ninth decade, and perhaps even beyond the ninth decade of life.[2] However, progressively increasing incidence with age is also associated with many other "normal" physical processes as well as with certain other pathological processes. For example, in men the prostate gland surrounding the urethra enlarges progressively with aging.[4] Analogously, the incidence of cancer of the large intestine increases with each decade of life in American men.[5] For men, we are less justified in declaring intellectual decline synonymous with old age than we are in making benign prostatic hypertrophy synonymous with old age.

Associating intellectual decline with "weakness" also obscures the true nature of senile and presenile dementia. There is no occurrence of physical weakness or debility in the sense of a loss of physical strength associated with the condition. Nonetheless, there is a form of weakness which occurs in brain failure, in that increased fatigue occurs in some persons with the condition. Even more important is the intellectual weakness which occurs in persons with severe brain failure. This intellectual weakness is best described by coining a new phrase to identify the symptoms, "cognitive abulia." "Abulia" is psychiatric terminology for "a loss or marked diminution of the will power."[6] Cognitive abulia is a form of intellectual weakness which commonly occurs in severe brain failure. Essentially, sufferers from it are incapable of maintaining a new thought or idea long enough to act upon it effectively. Hence they can't carry out or follow through on their decisions. This results in a form of intellectual weakness which is distinct from physical debility or loss of strength.

Brain failure, or age-associated loss of intellect, also needs to be distinguished from "infirmity of mind and body." Numerous mental disorders entirely unrelated to senility can be called, with equal justification, "infirmities of the mind." Schizophrenia, mania, depression, and alcohol intoxication are but a few examples of other "infirmities of the mind." Furthermore, neither brain failure nor any of the preceding examples are truly "infirmities of the mind and body." That phrase would more appropriately be applied to conditions that, like syphilis, truly affect both the brain and other organs.

The definition of senility found in *Webster's* would clearly appear to be inadequate to describe the condition which is the concern of this volume. The moment people identify a condition or a concept which they consider in any way significant, they give that concept a name. The condition which we shall be discussing in this book afflicts more than 1 million Americans (the very lowest estimate), and has been described as the fourth or fifth leading cause of death in the United States.[2,3] Yet among the several hundred thousand entries in the new *Webster's* there is no word which adequately describes this condition.

It is difficult to discuss a condition for which no word exists. Indeed, it is very easy for people to completely ignore or deny a condition which they do not even have a word for. Nevertheless, the illness we shall be discussing is not only widespread, it is increasing at a genuinely epidemic rate as the average longevity of peoples throughout the world increases. For convenience, throughout this book when we use the term "senility," we shall be using it in the very narrow sense of "an infirmity of the mind," and more precisely, "a specific type of infirmity of the mind which is frequently associated with aging." Using the word in this sense, the United States government recently released statistics which showed that senility afflicts 58 percent of the more than 1 million Americans in nursing homes, making it, according to the government health survey, the most common chronic illness to strike them.[*4] Of course, removing sufferers from the community and confining them to institutions makes it much easier for the community to ignore that condition. Indeed, not only are senile persons an absolute majority among residents of nursing homes, but vast numbers are confined within other chronic institutions such as mental hospitals. State mental hospitals and veterans hospitals in particular often have a large

---

* Arthritis or rheumatism ranked next on the list of chronic illnesses, plaguing 34.3 percent of nursing home residents, and heart ailments were third, with 33.5 percent of residents suffering from various chronic heart conditions.

proportion of senile patients. One source states that of the patients in state and county mental hospitals over the age of 65, more than half have the diagnosis of "senile dementia."[5] Despite these dramatic statistics, it is thought that at least half of moderately to severely impaired senile individuals remain within the community and either care for themselves as best they can or, more frequently, are assisted by their spouses, siblings, children, or other relatives. But man's capacity for denial of that which he would prefer not to face is such that one of the few books written for the general reader dealing specifically with this condition gainsays the threat, the magnitude, and even the present existence of senility. ". . . for the first time since man appeared on this planet, the terrifying shadow of the madness that man has learned to call senility has been lifted. At long last we can truly speak of the end of senility, and of the obsolescence, as well of 'old age' as we have always known it."[6]

How then do we explain all those people in the nursing homes and other institutions?

In the past two decades, medical scientists have ceased to ignore this area and have begun to make some progress in learning about and treating senility. It is this progress—the realistic achievements and the hope and future directions—which will be the major concern of this book.

Historically physicians have most frequently classified the syndrome of brain failure, which they frequently observed in their middle-aged and particularly in their elderly patients, as a "dementia," that is, a kind of "general mental 'deterioration.' "[7] Specifically, it has been referred to as "senile type dementia" when it has occurred in people over a certain age, generally 65 or older. This condition was described by Esquirol in 1838 in a French textbook of psychiatry in terms with which modern psychiatrists would not quarrel.[8] Esquirol described "démence sénile" as an illness in which there occurs a weakening of the memory for recent experiences and a loss of drive and willpower. The condition appears gradually and may be accompanied by emotional disturbances, he stated accurately. In 1906 Alois Alzheimer described a similar condition with the same symptoms developing in persons under the age of 65, a condition which has been named for him as "Alzheimer's disease." Another form of dementia generally occurring before the age of 65 and also with very similar symptoms was described by Arnold Pick in 1892 and came to be known as "Pick's disease." Together, Alzheimer's disease and the much less frequent disease described by Pick have come to be recognized as the "presenile dementias."

Much of medical science and practice is an arcane and scholarly discipline. Consequently, it is common for exceedingly rare and unusual conditions to receive as much attention in the medical literature and in medical research as much more frequently observed maladies. Fortunately, this approach, although certainly not the most sensible, often eventually yields dividends when the unusual conditions are found to tell us something useful about the more mundane illnesses. Nowhere is this process more evident than in the area of dementia. As we shall see later, one of the greatest breakthroughs in this field was made in a disease area which was so rare that cases had to be collected from all over the world, and the researchers, who eventually received a Nobel Prize in recognition of their discovery, published a public acknowledgment of every physician around the world who was kind enough to contribute a case.[9]

A similar process has occurred with regard to scientific interest in and investigation of what doctors called the senile and the presenile dementias. Dementia, occurring in the "senium," that is, the period after age 65, is of course very common. Although physicians have not been as negligent as laymen in that at least physicians have always had a word for this disorder, they have until very recently done very little more than name it. Once the diagnosis of senile dementia was made, neither clinicians nor researchers devoted much more time, effort, or thought to the condition. No doubt this lack of interest was merely one aspect of physicians' historic relative lack of knowledge of, interest in, and hope in the treatment of aging-related illness in general, which in turn was a product of societal prejudices against aged people in general.[10] The conditions of the "presenium," on the other hand, although uncommon, received at least as much interest and attention as the much more frequent later-onset condition. Because of this lack of proportion, a large amount of information has accumulated on Alzheimer's disease, which fortunately, as we shall see, tells us a great deal about senility.

A measure of the scientific neglect which senility has received until very recently can be obtained by reference to the standard medical texts. Among the medical disciplines, senile dementia has fallen primarily within the province of the specialties of psychiatry and neurology.

The standard American psychiatric text of the late 60s and early

70s is a huge tome comprising 1,666 pages. Only one-half of one of these pages is devoted to senile dementia, Alzheimer's disease, and Pick's disease combined.[11] The standard American neurology textbook from a later period, published in 1973, finds no space at all in its 841 pages for senile dementia, other than to mention its existence.[12] Indicative of the trend described above, however, we here find fully four pages of text and references on the presenile dementias. Between 1973 and 1975 a very fortuitous and important change occurred in medical thought. The 1975 edition of the standard psychiatric textbook (an even more massive compilation, this time comprising two volumes and 2,609 pages) finds two pages for senile dementia, which, however, are put under the heading "Senile Dementia (Alzheimer's Disease)."[13] What good fortune for physicians and scientists studying senility. Suddenly the relatively rare Alzheimer's disease, about which relatively so much information has accumulated, is being identified as the same entity as senile dementia.

Of course textbooks necessarily lag somewhat behind the vanguard of current research and thought. It has recently been proposed that the term "brain failure" replace "senile dementia" and "senility." "Progressive idiopathic dementia" and "primary degenerative dementia" are more descriptive terms. The latter has become the official terminology in the American diagnostic nomenclature.[14] Currently the various terms are used synonymously by scientists and medical researchers. In the remainder of this book we will follow this procedure and use the various terms interchangeably. Alzheimer's disease is not synonymous with senility as implied in that recent psychiatric text. It is, however, now thought to be the most important contributor to the syndrome* in a majority of senile people.

What finally got scientists and medical researchers to pay serious attention to senility? We have already mentioned the serendipitous finding that it had something to do with Alzheimer's disease, so that scientists were provided with a ready-made, previously painstakingly acquired body of knowledge regarding the condition. However, as is always true in scientific endeavor, social, economic, political, historical, and technological forces have contributed importantly to our newfound insight.

Although scientific and technological progress has not altered the

---

* A medical "syndrome" is a group of symptoms which commonly occur together but do not necessarily have the same origin.

human "lifespan," that is, the maximum age to which people can aspire to live, it has reduced many of the maladies which formerly struck down people in their youth or in middle age. The result has been that an increasingly greater proportion of the population is reaching old age.

This trend is of relatively recent origin. The human population has increased with increasing rapidity since about 1750. National registries of vital statistics provide concordant information from Sweden beginning in 1749, from France beginning in 1800, from England and Wales beginning in 1838, and from Ireland beginning in 1871. Birth rates have fallen fairly steadily, and, allowing for net migrations, the populations of Western nations have grown in spite of lower birth rates. For example, the population of England and Wales tripled between 1700 and 1851, and has very nearly tripled since then. The direct cause of the rise in population is the decline in mortality. Most of the decline has been due to the reduction of the effects of infectious disease. Until about 1900, there appears to have been no decrease in infant mortality or in mortality among those over 45. The increase in life expectancy appears to have come through the steady reduction at just those ages where mortality was naturally lowest, the years from 2 to 45. Since 1900, man has slowly succeeded in reducing mortality among those over 45 as well.[15] In 1900 only 4 percent of the population of the United States was over the age of 65. In the 1970 census, this proportion had grown to 10 percent of the population. There are now more than 10 million Americans over 73 years of age, and 1 million have reached the age of 85. Dr. Robert N. Butler has dramatized the political significance of this demographic shift: "Older people constitute 10 percent of the population, but they represent 15 percent of eligible voters. In addition, they have a better voting record than do almost any other age group. Ninety percent are registered to vote and over 65 percent of these vote regularly."[16]

One result of the political and medical fallout from the increased number of aged persons was that a White House conference on aging, held in 1967, eventually led to the establishment of a National Institute of Aging within the National Institutes of Health. Dr. Butler, a psychiatrist, was appointed the first director of the new National Institute of Aging. From this source and from others, also of recent origin, have come funds, which are for the first time being made readily available for research into the age-related illnesses.

A number of recent technological innovations either have stimulated interest in and research into senility or promise to contribute in important ways to our understanding of the condition within the next few years. An example of the former is the hyperbaric (increased pressure) chamber. This device can be used to immerse a person in atmospheric or other gases at increased pressures. It is commonly used to repressurize deep-sea divers who have ascended too rapidly to prevent them from developing "the bends." Knowing that the brains of senile persons utilize less oxygen than those of nonsenile people of the same age, researchers reasoned that supplying the brain with increased amounts of oxygen under increased pressure might reverse the condition. The initial scientific report on this treatment was very favorable and appeared in the *New England Journal of Medicine,* a very widely read and prestigious medical journal.[17] It resulted in widespread investigation of this treatment and greatly increased interest in senility. If the treatment was to be accepted as effective, then scientists had to develop measures which could be used to prove or disprove its efficacy. A wide variety of such measures were indeed developed, some of which will be described subsequently. The controversy over the true value of hyperbaric treatment in senility lasted for most of a decade and resulted in the establishment of subgroups within the major psychiatric research centers which developed particular expertise in the evaluation and treatment of senility. One such subgroup became the Geriatric Study Program at the Millhauser Laboratories of the New York University Medical Center. Similar groups developed in Boston, Houston, and a few other centers. My associates in New York, in collaboration with researchers at the National Institute of Mental Health, eventually performed the definitive study which demonstrated that hyperbaric treatment was not of significant value in the treatment of senility.[18] This study was published in January 1978, by which time a very large amount of information about brain failure had accumulated.

Another technological breakthrough is our recently developed ability to measure the flow of blood through the brain. This technique and related, even more sophisticated measures promise to genuinely increase our understanding of the effects of aging and senility on the brain.

The average blood flow in the human brain was first determined in 1944 by Seymour S. Kety, a psychiatrist who has become famous for his research into this and other areas. His technique has since been improved upon to such an extent that it is now possible to measure the amount of blood flowing through different areas of the brain and to observe changes in blood flow depending upon the tasks with which the mind is occupied.[19] Hence we can now tell to which areas of the brain the blood flows when we are sleeping and to which areas of the brain blood tends to go when we are awake. Even more significantly, it has been found that when we hear sounds, the blood tends to go to areas of the brain which are known to be "hearing centers," and when we open our eyes, blood flow increases to "visual centers" of the brain. Since the blood flow in the brain is shifted to those areas where it is most needed, by measuring blood flow, we can tell which areas of the brain are healthy and working and which are weakened or dead.

In senile people parts of the brain often decay (the technical word for this is "atrophy"). Other parts of the brain function with varying degrees of effectiveness. The location of areas of weakening or decay in the brain can tell physicians something about what the cause or causes of the brain failure are, and which treatment or treatments would be most useful. On the other hand, the effectiveness of a new treatment can be more sensitively determined by finding whether it increases blood flow to certain brain areas, as well as to the brain as a whole. Several kinds of drugs which have been found to cause an increase in the blood flow to the brain are currently being investigated in the treatment of senility, and at least some of those compounds appear particularly promising at this time.

In collaboration with scientists at the Brookhaven National Laboratories and with other scientists at the New York University Medical Center, we at the Geriatric Study Program are currently developing new methods for distinguishing healthy areas of the brain from decayed areas. One such method measures the health and functioning of an area by the amount of sugar it uses for energy. Dead tissue, of course, uses no sugar, and active brain tissue requires more sugar for its actions than weakened brain tissue. Another method which we are investigating uses a computer to give us even more information about the flow of blood to different areas of the brain.

Computers have already revolutionized the kinds of X-ray pictures we can take of the brain. Conventional X-rays, the kind that doctors use to tell whether a bone is broken, only give us pictures of "hard tissues," such as bones and teeth. A conventional X-ray does not show the brain at all, only the skull. By injecting radioactive substances into the blood circulation, doctors became able to take pictures of the brain itself. In the 1970s this technique was improved enormously by using a computer to "reconstruct" pictures of the brain based upon the flow of radioactive substances through the tissues of the brain. This new method, which is both simple and safe, is called "computerized axial tomographic scanning" or "CAT scans" for short. CAT scans are currently being done at more than 1,000 centers around the world. By looking at a CAT scan, a doctor can tell which areas of the brain have decayed and whether certain serious conditions are present which may account for the decay. Researchers are currently relating these pictures of brain decay to the amount and kinds of memory loss and thinking impairment which senile people experience. The pictures are being used to improve our diagnosis of the specific causes of brain failure and to improve our predictions regarding its long-term outlook.

History, politics, science, and technology have converged to bring about a new discovery of senility in the last half of the twentieth century. Out of this discovery has come a burgeoning of knowledge and of hope. What follows is a description of that knowledge and of our realistic hopes and expectations for the successful treatment of senile dementia in the near future.

Notes

1. *Webster's New Twentieth Century Dictionary,* unabridged, 2d ed., William Collins and World Publishing Co., Inc., 1975, p. 1651.
2. Angel, R. W., Understanding and diagnosing senile dementia. *Geriatrics,* August 1977, pp. 47–49.
3. Katzman, R., and Karasu, T. B., Differential diagnosis of dementia. In *Neurological and Sensory Disorders in the Elderly,* ed. by W. S. Fields, Stratton Intercontinental Medical Book Corp., New York, 1975, pp. 103–134.
4. National Center of Health Statistics, survey conducted 1973–74, reported 1978.
5. Riley, M. W., and Foner, A., *Aging and Society,* Russell Sage Foundation, New York, 1968.
6. Freese, A. S., *The End of Senility,* Arbor House, New York, 1978, p. xi.
7. *Stedman's Medical Dictionary,* 21st ed., Williams & Wilkins Company, Baltimore, 1966, p. 421.
8. Esquirol, J. E. D., *Des Maladies Mentales,* Balliere, Paris, 1838.
9. Traub, R., Gajdusek, D. C., and Gibbs, C. J., Jr., Transmissible virus dementia: The relation of transmissible spongiform encephalopathy to Creutzfeldt-Jakob disease. In *Aging and Dementia,* ed. by L. Smith and M. Kinsbourne, Spectrum Publications, Inc., New York, 1977, Appendix 1, pp. 147–154.

10. See Butler, R. N., *Why Survive? Being Old in America,* Harper & Row, 1975, for a more complete discussion of this.
11. Freedman, A. M., and Kaplan, H. I., (eds.), *Comprehensive Textbook of Psychiatry,* Williams & Wilkins Company, Baltimore, 1967, p. 460.
12. Merritt, H. H., *A Textbook of Neurology,* Lea & Febiger, Philadelphia, 5th ed., 1973, pp. 442–445.
13. Freedman, A. M., Kaplan, H. I., and Sadock, B. J., *Comprehensive Textbook of Psychiatry,* 2d ed., Williams & Wilkins Company, Baltimore, 1975, pp. 1086–1087.
14. American Psychiatric Association, *Diagnostic and Statistical Manual of Mental Disorders,* 3d ed. (*DSM = III*), 1980.
15. McKeown, Thomas, *The Modern Rise of Population,* Academic Press, New York, 1976.
16. Butler, op. cit., p. 324.
17. Jacobs, E., Winter, P. M., Alvis, H. J., et al., Hyperoxygenation effects on cognitive functioning in the aged. *New England J. Med.* 281: 753, 1969.
18. Raskin, A., Gershon, S., Crook, T. H., Sathananthan, G., and Ferris, S., The effects of hyperbaric and normabaric oxygen on cognitive impairment in the elderly. *Arch. Gen. Psychiat.* 35: 50–56, 1978.
19. Lassen, N. A., Ingvar, D. H. and Skinhøj, E., Brain functions and blood flow. *Scientific American,* October 1978, pp. 62–71.

Chapter 2

Plaques and Tangles: Understanding Alzheimer's Disease

LAYMEN AND INDEED MOST PHYSICIANS still think of "hardening of the arteries," or arteriosclerosis, as being responsible for most instances of senility. The popular image is of blood vessels which become progressively narrowed from fatty deposits. As the vessels of the brain become strangulated and sclerosed, less and less blood is able to reach the brain and provide the nourishment necessary for optimal functioning. Behavioral deterioration is thought to result from these circulatory changes. First, a person may begin to forget things. Later, the lack of blood and oxygen may cause the person to become entirely demented. Often the narrowing of the blood vessels is thought to result in strokes and, ultimately, in death. In the words of a modern textbook of pathology, "ischemic damage to the heart, brain and kidneys, caused by atherosclerosis,* accounts today for approximately one-half of all deaths in the United States and Great Britain."[1]

As is probably true of all myths, medical and otherwise, a germ of

---

* "Arteriosclerosis" literally means "hardening of the arteries," but more accurately it refers to a group of processes which have in common thickening and loss of elasticity of arterial walls. "Atherosclerosis" is characterized by the formation of fatty deposits in the walls of the arteries. Atherosclerosis is the most common form of arteriosclerosis and is the form most commonly referred to.

truth gave credence to these conceptions. Arteriosclerotic changes in the walls of blood vessels and in the diameter of blood vessels do occur. Also, these changes are encountered more frequently as persons age. They do cause narrowing of the coronary arteries, and arteriosclerosis has been shown to be strongly associated with heart attacks and many forms of heart disease. Because of the age relationship observed with respect to arteriosclerotic deposits, "senile" (in the sense of age-related!) deterioration of the walls of arteries, leading to arteriosclerosis, is said to occur.

Association does not imply causation. For example, graying of the hair and wrinkling of the skin are definitely associated with aging. Brain failure is definitely associated with aging as well. It does not follow that gray hair causes brain failure! Neither, for that matter, does it follow that brain failure causes gray hair. It was this kind of simple error of logic, together with the image of narrowed cerebral blood vessels and the resultant decrease in blood flow, which satisfied virtually all physicians and laymen that arteriosclerosis caused senility. As we have seen, the subject was rarely examined in great detail anyway. Repetition caused the myth to strengthen.

Other myths have sprung up concerning atherosclerosis, based upon similar combinations of "common sense" (unfortunately, all too often "common sense" becomes synonymous with "faulty logic") and scanty evidence. A recent example is the myth that marathon runners do not have coronary atherosclerosis.[2] It is known that active persons have less coronary atherosclerosis than their inactive counterparts. An autopsy was done on a single marathon runner and only minimal coronary atherosclerosis was found.[3] Based upon these two truths, a myth arose that marathon runners are immune to coronary atherosclerosis.[4,5]

There are several errors in rushing to this conclusion. Although more active persons have less atherosclerosis, it does not follow that activity is the cause of this phenomenon. For example, active persons may be thinner and smoke less, and be less likely to develop the fatty deposits for those reasons. Also, it is an error to make universal generalizations from one observation. Just because one marathon runner did not have marked coronary atherosclerosis, it does not follow that all marathon runners do not. Indeed, when autopsies were eventually done on other marathon runners, some were found to *have* coronary atherosclerosis of the same magnitude as that observed in many nonrunners.[6]

In the 1960s some disturbing facts accumulated which the myth of the atherosclerotic origin of senile dementia was unable to explain. Some English pathologists examined the blood vessels of persons who had died with dementia and compared them with the blood vessels of persons who were not demented at the time of their demise.[7] They examined not only the vessels of the brain but those of the entire body. They found roughly the same arteriosclerotic changes in the demented and the nondemented groups! Another team of pathologists repeated their work, examining the brains of over 100 patients, and confirmed that arteriosclerotic changes appeared no greater in the brains of demented and, presumably, mostly senile persons.[8]

Subsequently, an English group of pathologists and psychiatrists finally set out to determine what changes genuinely occurred in persons with dementia. Their work has revolutionized our thinking in regard to this major illness and has virtually launched the scientific investigation of senile dementia. Tomlinson, Blessed, and Roth undertook a series of investigations in which they examined the brains of demented persons.[9,10,11,12] Fifty demented individuals over the age of 65 were followed during their lifetimes. When these persons died, their brains were autopsied. Comparisons were made with findings in the brains of 28 nondemented, elderly control subjects.

More than 50 percent of the demented persons had pathological findings indicative of Alzheimer's disease (see Table 2–1). This was at the time known as Alzheimer's type, presenile dementia, and *by defini-*

T A B L E 2–1.   Modern Classification of Senile Dementia

I.   S.D.A.T.
    Senile dementia Alzheimer's type or
    Alzheimer's disease or
    Progressive idiopathic dementia
      More than 50% of autopsied cases

II. M.I.D.
    Multi-infarct dementia or
    Dementia secondary to stroke and cardiovascular disease
      Approximately 15% of autopsied cases

III. Mixed
    Dementia secondary to S.D.A.T. + M.I.D.
      Approximately 25% of autopsied cases

IV. Other
    e.g., "Pseudodementia" secondary to depression
      Approximately 10% of total

tion was said not to occur in elderly persons. This definition has subsequently been broadened so that "Alzheimer's disease" now refers to a characteristic set of pathological findings rather than only to that characteristic pathology coming from a restricted age group. Hence, "Alzheimer's disease" is now thought to be the same condition whether it occurs in a forty-five-year-old person or a ninety-five-year-old person. The underlying pathology and the disease process, so far as is known, is the same, regardless of the age of onset. Nevertheless, the traditional distinction among Alzheimer's disease of presenile onset versus senile dementia of the Alzheimer's type (S.D.A.T.) is occasionally made. This need not be confusing, if we recognize that the disease process remains fundamentally the same whenever it finds expression throughout the human life span.

These pathological findings, coming as they did from a group of distinguished medical investigators, genuinely sounded the death knell of the arteriosclerotic theories of the origins of the senile dementia so commonly observed with aging. Nevertheless, such is the power of myth and popular belief that although the work of Tomlinson and his colleagues was completed in the 60s, it was not until 1974 that an "official" refutation of those theories was promulgated. Three prominent scientists from three countries and two continents joined in a paper in the *Lancet,* the prestigious British medical journal. They declared that "the use of the term 'cerebral atherosclerosis' to describe mental deterioration in the elderly is probably the most common medical misdiagnosis."[13] They went on to describe a new theory of how conditions affecting the blood vessels may contribute to senile dementia in a minority of cases. More about that later. Most importantly, they declared that they considered the Alzheimer changes seen by Tomlinson and his colleagues the causative factor in a majority of persons with senile dementia. The medical and scientific communities have been adapting to these changing conceptualizations ever since. Such is the power of tradition that, as of this writing, the statement that "the use of the term 'cerebral atherosclerosis' to describe mental deterioration in the elderly is probably the most common medical misdiagnosis," undoubtedly remains correct. The vast majority of professional and lay persons have never even heard of this "Alzheimer's disease" which is now thought to be so crucial to the origins and evolution of senile dementia. Everyone, of course, is familiar with the progressive mental changes which are so commonly observed in aged persons.

What is Alzheimer's disease?

In the first decade of this century, Alois Alzheimer described a disease of middle life in which there is progressive deterioration of behavior. In the original patient described by Alzheimer, the first evidence of disease was progressive jealousy.[14] Paranoid traits and other major behavioral disturbances, in addition to disturbances of memory and intellect, have ever since been frequently mentioned as part of the disease. Seizures are often mentioned as occurring in the later stages of the illness. Eventually all higher brain functions are thought to be lost. Accompanying these mental changes are physical changes in the brain substance itself. The substance of the brain decays, particularly the outer, or cortical, layers. The brain decay is most severe in the area of the forehead (frontal) and inside the temples (temporal) (see Figure 2-1). Eventually the entire outer brain substance decays. Death was traditionally said to occur from two to ten years after the onset of the process.

The clinical descriptions of Alzheimer's deterioration were probably based upon observations of persons whose illness was already severely advanced. The clinical course of the illness will be described subsequently in greater detail. However, the descriptions of the gross changes in the brain substance remain current. The hallmarks of these changes are those pathological findings which can be observed under the microscope. It is these pathological findings which provide the

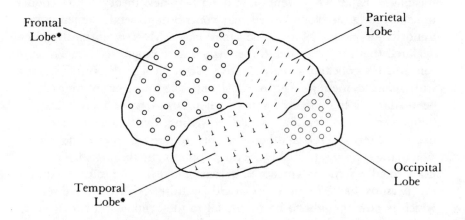

*Major loci of pathology in Alzheimer's disease

Figure 2.1.   The Outer Portions of the Brain (the Cerebral Cortex)

clues to the origins of Alzheimer's disease and to the majority of senile dementias which are now known to result from this illness.

What are the pathological changes in Alzheimer's disease? Three important kinds of brain changes occur. They are *neurofibrillary tangles, senile plaques,* and *granulovacuolar degeneration.* The most important and characteristic change is the appearance of unusual quantities of neurofibrils in certain areas of the brain. These neurofibrils have a characteristic shape and size. In Alzheimer's disease they are found predominantly in the cerebral cortex. They are found in particularly large concentration in the hippocampus (see Figure 2-2), which is the part of the brain thought to be associated with short-term memory, and especially in the pyramidal cells of the hippocampus.[12] They can be readily identified by neuropathologists using silver-staining techniques. Some degree of neurofibrillary tangle formation occurs in the hippocampus and the amygdaloid nucleus of many middle-aged and elderly people. The incidence of the tangles in the brains of persons without evidence of dementia appears to increase with age, so that virtually all examined brains of persons over 90 years of age show some tangle formation. In Alzheimer's disease, however, the density and distribution of these tangles are markedly increased. In the study of Tomlinson, Blessed, and Roth the quantity of tangles in the brain tissue was estimated on a four-point scale from none to numerous. Of the 28 control patients who were without symptoms of dementia, 90 percent did not show *any* neurofibrillary tangle formation in the neocortex. The remaining control patients showed a few scattered tangles. In contrast, all of the demented patients who were diagnosed pathologically as suffering from Alzheimer's disease had moderate to numerous quantities of neurofibrillary tangles scattered throughout the neocortex.

The neurofibrillary tangles found in Alzheimer's disease are now known to consist of pairs of filaments wrapped around each other in a helical fashion. The configuration is consistent, and the helix is said to show periodicity, narrowing to a width of 100 Å at intervals of approximately 800 Å [15,16] (see Figure 2-3A). the tangles are located within the neuron, most frequently in the area surrounding the nucleus but also to some extent within the neuronal processes (axons and dendrites).

Tomlinson, in an update of his earlier work, has stated that "in the study of more than 120 cases of assessed old individuals, large numbers of neurofibrillary tangles throughout the neocortex have invariably been associated with dementia."[17] Interestingly, although the

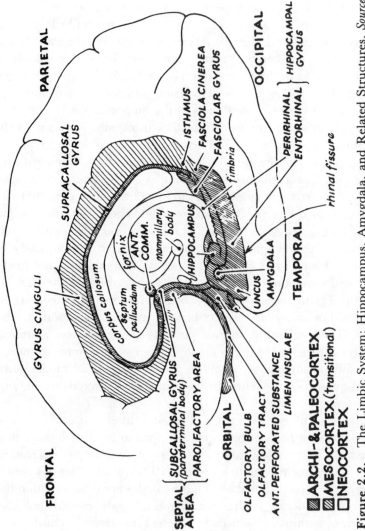

Figure 2.2. The Limbic System: Hippocampus, Amygdala, and Related Structures. *Source: Louis Hausman, Illustrations of the Nervous System, Atlas III, 1961, fig. 83, p. 94. Courtesy of Charles Thomas, Publisher, Springfield, Illinois.*

A. Schematic View

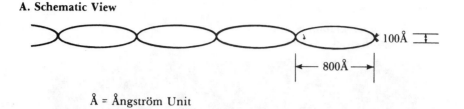

Å = Ångström Unit

1 Ångström Unit = 1/10000 micron = 0.0000001 mm. =
        1/254000000 in.

Figure 2.3.   Alzheimer's Neurofibrillary Tangles (Paired Helical Filaments, or PHFs)

Alzheimer's-type neurofibrillary tangles, which are also known as paired helical filaments (PHFs) because of their unique configuration, have been found only in human beings, they are encountered in certain human conditions apart from Alzheimer's disease (see Table 2-2). For example, persons with Down's syndrome who survive into adulthood frequently develop a dementia in which PHFs are present in great abundance in the brain. Down's syndrome, commonly known as mongolism, is a genetic abnormality which is generally characterized by the presence of an extra chromosome.

PHFs are also present in other dementias of quite different origin. For example, dementia pugilistica, commonly known as "punch-drunkenness," is a generalized mental disturbance resulting from

TABLE 2-2.   **Conditions with Neurofibrillary Tangles**

Condition	Location
Alzheimer's disease	Throughout the neocortex and hippocampus
Normal aging	Throughout the neocortex, hippocampus, and amygdala
Down's syndrome (mongolism)	Throughout the neocortex
Dementia pugilistica (punch-drunkenness)	Substantia nigra
Parkinsonian-dementia complex of Guam	Substantia nigra
Postencephalitic Parkinsonism	Substantia nigra
Related but different structures in aging rhesus monkeys	

B. Electronmicrographic Sketch
  (Magnification × 125,000).

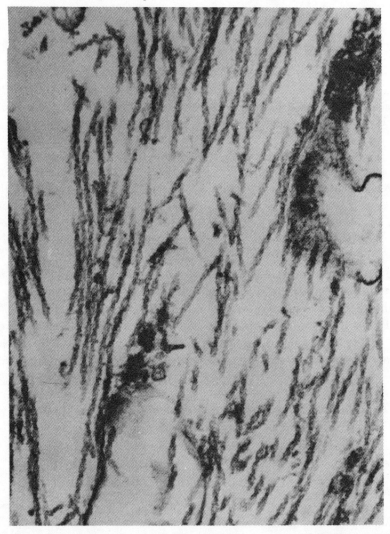

Figure 2.3, cont. A paired-helical-filament-enriched fraction prepared from a case of Alzheimer's dementia. *Source: "Neurofibrillary Pathology," by K. Igbal, H. M. Wisniewski, I. Grundke-Iqbal, and R. D. Terry, in* The Aging Brain and Senile Dementia, Advances in Behavioral Biology, *Kalidas Nandy and Ira Sherwin* (eds)., *Vol. 23, 1977, p. 218, Plenum Press, New York and London. Reproduced with permission.*

repeated head trauma. It was originally observed among experienced boxers, who sometimes developed a tendency to be unsteady on their feet, to be forgetful, and to be slow in their thinking and movement in general.[18] PHFs are found in this condition.

They are also found in certain forms of Parkinson's disease, notably postencephalitic Parkinsonism and the so-called Parkinsonian-dementia complex of Guam.

Both of these conditions are interesting. Postencephalitic Parkinsonism exists primarily as a sequela of the post-World War I flu epidemic. Many of the millions of persons who succumbed to the influenza developed an encephalitic* condition which was characterized by long periods of sleep. Hence this encephalitis became known as "encephalitis lethargica." It has been discovered that very many of the persons who develop Parkinsonism today are survivors of that influenza epidemic who developed the encephalitic complication. The same neurofibrillary tangles which are so characteristic of Alzheimer's disease are found in the brains of persons with this Parkinsonian condition which is seemingly of viral causation.

Hence we can find tangles identical to those characteristic of Alzheimer's disease, the major cause of senility, in persons with a dementia related to a chromosomal abnormality, namely mongolism, and in the brains of persons with a dementia related to injury, dementia pugilistica, and the tangles are present in the postencephalitic Parkinsonian condition of possible viral origin. And to this list of seemingly diverse causes must be added another—genetic. The Parkinsonian-dementia complex of Guam is a rare inherited condition which is found only among the Chamorro people of that island. Those who succumb to this rare condition develop both Parkinsonism and generalized mental deterioration (dementia). They have neurofibrillary tangles present in their brains in great abundance.

What are these neurofibrillary tangles, or PHFs? No one really knows. There are certain normal intracellular structures known as neurofilaments and neurotubules which may be related to the pathological development of tangles, but this has not been proven. It is known that some neurological diseases produce neurofibrillary tangles which differ from those seen in Alzheimer's disease. It is also known that although Alzheimer's type tangles are only found in human be-

---

* An "encephalitis" is a condition in which there is a generalized inflammation of the substance of the brain.

ings, similar structures with a periodicity half that found naturally in human PHFs have been observed in aged rhesus monkeys.[19]

What is the significance of the neurofibrillary tangles found in the brain in such great abundance in Alzheimer's type dementia and in the other conditions described above? A number of clues emerge. In consideration of the variety of conditions in which the tangles may be observed, it would appear that chemical and/or physical trauma to the brain of diverse origin might result in a common end process which leads to the tangle formation. The data provide a number of intriguing leads, but before pursuing these, something needs to be said about the location of the tangles in the different conditions.

We have said that relatively small concentrations of the tangles are observed with increasing frequency as successively older groups of persons are studied. These tangles occur in the parts of the brain known as the hippocampus and the amygdaloid nucleus. Both of these structures are constituents of what is known as the "limbic system" of the brain (see Figure 2-2). The "limbic system" is an interconnecting network of nuclei and tracts. It can be viewed as a closed circuit that permits the projection of impulses to and from the higher cortical centers. It is often described as the "seat of emotion" in the brain. As described by Papez in 1937, emotion is not a mystical entity, but "a physiologic process which depends on an anatomic mechanism."[20] The anatomic mechanism he identified as the limbic system, which also became known as "Papez' circuit."

Apart from being constituents of this brain circuit thought to be the seat of the emotions, the hippocampus and the amygdala are thought to have functions of their own. Bilateral damage to the hippocampus results in permanent arrest of recent memory. People with these lesions are unable to register any new memories. Although they retain memory for events prior to the trauma, for new events all recollections disappear within minutes after their occurrence. This happens despite the continued ability of the people to pay attention to the new material.

Injuries in the amygdala, which is really a series of nuclei (nerve centers) in the temporal lobe of the brain, also produce dramatic changes in behavior. Removal of the amygdalae of dominant male monkeys transformed them into submissive animals.[21] Monkeys become not only submissive but placid and pathologically lacking in fear. For example, monkeys which ordinarily show a healthy fear of snakes will play with them and even eat them![22] Amygdalectomy has succeeded in reducing aggression in some people with severe rage and aggression.[23]

Hence we can reasonably postulate that the tangles often seen under an ordinary light microscope in the hippocampus and amygdala in aged persons may be related to certain memory and behavioral changes which occur in some elderly people. Not everyone who lives beyond the seventh decade suffers from memory deficit, but those who do suffer from it often display a deficit of short-term memory as the earliest symptom. This is certainly compatible with minor trauma concentrated in the hippocampal area. Many elderly people with early symptoms of memory impairment also exhibit what is referred to in psychiatric terminology as "a flat affect." This means there is a paucity of emotional response underlying their actions. The potentially devastating impact of their incipient loss of memory, in particular, is accepted with equanimity. Their relatively shallow emotional responses are compatible with the kinds of deficits described after damage to the amygdala.

In Alzheimer's disease, the tangles are seen in highest concentration in the hippocampus but are observed to a lesser extent throughout the neocortex, the outer layer of the brain. These observations would explain some of the most notable behavioral deficits in Alzheimer's sufferers, namely the memory deficit, particularly the loss of short-term memory, and the generalized dementia.

Persons with Down's syndrome who survive into the early decades of adult life often develop a dementia with senile features. Examination of the brain reveals a tangle distribution much like that of Alzheimer's. As we shall see, there are also other interrelationships between Down's syndrome and Alzheimer's disease, and knowledge of the former may increase our understanding of the latter.

Parkinsonism is a syndrome in which movements become slowed and the body becomes rigid. The slowing of movement and rigidity result in the shuffling gait which is one major characteristic of the syndrome. Another result of the muscular rigidity is an inability to adequately clear oral secretions and the consequent accumulation of saliva, leading to drooling. The syndrome's appearance alone suggests a dementia-like process, and the motoric impairment may result in impaired performance on certain psychological tests. Nevertheless, a true dementia is often seen accompanying a Parkinsonian state (see Chapter 4).

The pathology behind the Parkinsonian syndrome is known. There is a part of the brain which is ordinarily pigmented and has therefore been named the "substantia nigra" ("nigra" means "black"; hence, literally, "the black substance"). In Parkinsonian syndromes, this part of the brain loses its color. One of the great modern medical discoveries has been the determination of the causes of Parkinsonian changes. An important chemical in the brain known as "dopamine" has been found to be depleted in many parts of the brains of Parkinsonian patients.[24] If physicians administer a related compound, L-dopa, which is converted to dopamine in the body, many of the Parkinsonian symptoms improve dramatically. We now believe dopamine to be one of the basic "neurotransmitter" compounds. That is, we believe it to be a substance which communicates messages between nerves in certain parts of the brain.

As mentioned, tangles have been observed in certain Parkinsonian conditions, specifically in postencephalitic Parkinsonism and in the Parkinsonian-dementia complex of Guam. Dementia pugilistica, another condition in which tangles are commonly found, also includes a Parkinsonian syndrome as one of its common constituents. In all of these Parkinsonian syndromes with neurofibrillary tangle pathology, the tangles are found in particularly high concentration within the substantia nigra, the very part of the brain which is the primary locus of the Parkinsonian pathology!

The possible chemical interrelationship between Parkinsonian conditions and senility will be discussed later. For now we can say that the tangles of Alzheimer's disease, Down's syndrome, and "normal aging" are particularly clustered in certain regions, centering on the cortex and hippocampus, and that those of the Parkinsonian syndromes of diverse etiology center on the substantia nigra. In both cases the tangles appear to center on the brain regions which are primarily associated with the neurological impairment.

There is another important place where neurofibrillary tangles are found—in the area around senile plaques. As mentioned, these are the second major brain finding in Alzheimer's disease. Classical senile or neuritic plaques, as they are also called, consist of an amyloid core surrounded by degenerative neuronal processes and reactive nonneuronal cells. The degenerative neuronal processes are known to consist almost entirely of axonal terminals or perterminals. In the region of these degenerative neuronal processes, and to a lesser extent in the dendrites and synaptic endings outside the plaque area, one encounters the PHFs.

Plaques provide another link in our understanding of Alzheimer's disease and memory loss with aging. Like the tangles, increased concentrations of plaques are associated with dementia (see Figure 2-4). Also, just as tangles are found increasingly frequently in older populations, plaques are found more frequently as progressively older populations are studied. Plaques and tangles are commonly seen together in the brains of dements; that is, they tend to be found in the same general areas of the brain, and they tend to occur together in the same individuals. Uncommonly, however, examination of the brain of a demented person may reveal the presence of tangles in the absence of significant plaque formation, or vice versa. Unlike tangles, classical senile plaques apparently identical to those observed in humans have been discovered in animals.

The amyloid material which forms the core of senile plaques probably provides the key to their origin. Two kinds of amyloid material are known to occur. One kind is of unknown origin, although it is known to consist of protein material. The other form is thought to be a complex of immunoglobulin chains. Immunoglobulins are protein antibodies which organisms manufacture in response to antigenic material (a foreign protein, such as a virus, is a classical antigen). The plaques observed in senile dementia are thought to consist of this latter form of amyloid. It has been proposed that the plaques are formed when antigen-antibody complexes are ingested by white blood cells (phagocytes).[25,26] The complexes may be digested within the phagocytes, and the product may result in amyloid formation. Senile plaques are sometimes said to be located in the region of blood vessels. Accordingly, some scientists have theorized that the plaques result when the digested antigen-antibody complexes in the form of amyloid are released from the phagocytes ("phago" means "to eat" and "cytes" means "cells," ergo "cells which eat") and leak out through the blood vessels.

Further insight into the origin of the plaques and perhaps of senility itself is provided by an examination of the other conditions in both animals and man in which plaques have been found to occur (see Table 2-3). Dementia, as we shall see, has origins as diverse as the field of medicine itself. Some startling findings have recently been obtained about a small group of dementias. These findings collectively constitute one of the most exciting stories in modern medicine and seem to lead us directly to the doorstep of Alzheimer's disease itself.

Kuru, or "trembling with fear," is a progressive neurological

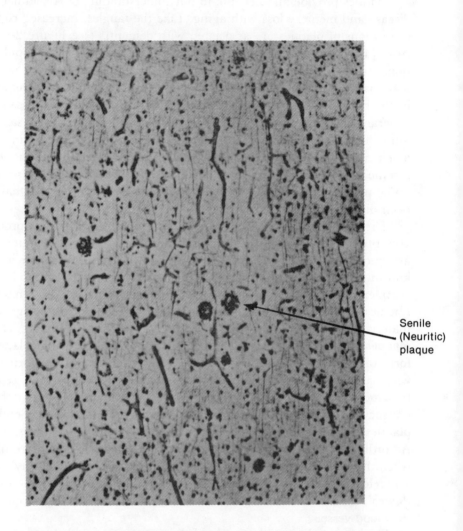

Senile
(Neuritic)
plaque

Appearance of senile plaques at around 8 per low-power field in the cortex
of a nondemented subject. (Counts performed on circular fields) von Braunmuhl × 88

Figure 2.4A.　Senile (Neuritic) Plaques. Low concentration—nondemented
subject. *Source: "Morphological Changes and Dementia in Old Age," by B. E.
Tomlinson, in* Aging and Dementia, *W. Lynn Smith and Marcel Kinsbourne (eds.),
Fig. 2, p. 31. Copyright 1977, Spectrum Publications, Inc., New York. Reproduced
with permission.*

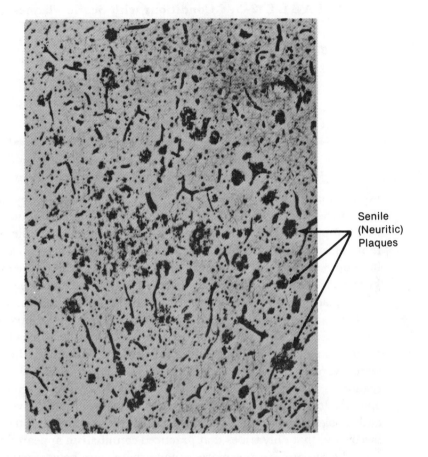

Senile
(Neuritic)
Plaques

Appearance of senile plaques in a field containing 62 from a
demented subject. In several places plaques are aggregated into
large masses. von Braunmuhl × 88

Figure 2.4B. Senile Plaques, cont. High concentration—demented subject. *Source: ''Morphological Changes and Dementia in Old Age,'' by B. E. Tomlinson, in* Aging and Dementia, *W. Lynn Smith and Marcel Kinsbourne (eds.), Fig. 3, p. 32. Copyright 1977, Spectrum Publications, Inc., New York. Reproduced with permission.*

disorder invariably ending in death. It is only known to occur among certain tribes in the highlands of New Guinea. Persons developing kuru begin to have difficulty walking. Subsequently they develop a hand tremor and their speech becomes slurred. They develop involuntary jerky movements and wormlike movements. They become cross-

T A B L E 2-3. Conditions with Senile Plaques

1. Alzheimer's disease
2. Down's syndrome
3. Normal aging
   a. Humans
   b. Dogs
4. Transmissible virus dementias
   a. Scrapie (in sheep)
   b. Mink encephalopathy
   c. Kuru (in man)
   d. Creutzfeldt-Jakob disease (in man and other primates)

eyed. Finally their thinking capacity begins to fade—they become demented. Within four months to two years of the appearance of the first symptoms, they invariably die. Most commonly they die of common infections which afflict those who are bed-ridden and weak. They develop bed sores which become infected, or they die of pneumonia. When one examines the brains of these unfortunate victims, one finds widespread loss of neurons and axons and amyloid plaques.[27]

For many years the origin of kuru remained mysterious. It was known to occur only in certain tribes and not in other tribes living in adjacent areas. Also, 80 percent of the adults afflicted with the disease were women. Children appeared to be about equally affected, regardless of sex. Physicians were at a loss to explain this epidemiologic distribution. The mystery was eventually solved by an anthropologist who lived among and studied these highland tribes. He discovered that only tribes that practiced cannibalism appeared to contract the disease. Furthermore, among these cannibalistic tribes, only those who cooked and ate the brains of their victims were susceptible. Why the peculiar sex incidence? In most tribes, he observed, ordinarily only the women and children ate the brains—the men ate the other body parts!

These discoveries appeared to explain the peculiar distribution of kuru, but what was the substance in the brain which caused the terrible "trembling with fear?" Whatever it was appeared to have very delayed effects because people were known to develop the first symptoms of kuru years after they had last dined on brain. It was natural to consider the possibility that some kind of infectious agent was transmitted in the brain material. However, an infectious disease would be expected to occur days or weeks following exposure, but kuru, as we said, developed years after the ingestion of the brain material.

The next clue to the origins of kuru came from studies of another closely similar disease found naturally in sheep and goats, known as scrapie. Like kuru, scrapie is a progressive, fatal neurological disease. Pathologically, the findings in the brains of the animals are very similar to those in the brains of people with kuru. Scrapie was first transmitted by researchers by inoculation of a ewe in 1899.[28] Many years later, it was shown that the infectious agent could pass through a fine filter and had other virus-like properties.[29] In 1961 scrapie was transmitted by inoculation into mice.[30] The mice developed a neurological disease very much like that occurring in the sheep. Apparently, genetic factors play a major role in determining the manner in which scrapie expresses itself, since different strains of mice have quite different incubation periods and clinical manifestations of illness, and the pathological findings vary in nature and distribution when the brain tissues from different strains are examined. In the 1970s it was shown that specific scrapie agents in certain strains of mice can induce senile plaque formation.[31,32] In certain mouse strains, plaques were seen in over 70 percent of the brains of mice with the clinical disease, but not in a large number of aged control mice. Just as in Alzheimer's senile dementia, some of the plaques in scrapie consist of amyloid fibers, degenerating neuronal processes, and reactive cells. It was also discovered that senile plaques could be found in the brains of minks which had contracted a neurological illness known as mink encephalopathy. Further investigations indicated that the mink appeared to contract the dementia from eating the carcasses of sheep infected with scrapie!

The infectious agent causing scrapie and mink encephalopathy has been termed a "slow virus" because of the long incubation period prior to the appearance of symptoms and the subsequent slowly progressing inexorable course of the disease. Might kuru, the human dementia which is so similar in course and pathology to these animal dementias, also be due to a slow virus? To prove that this was indeed the case, scientists would have to succeed in injecting an extract of brain material from a person infected with kuru into another organism and produce an illness resembling kuru itself. If the infectious agent were a virus, then the injectible extract would have to be filterable; that is, it would have to be able to pass through fine filters which would not permit relatively large infectious organisms such as bacteria to pass through. In 1965 Gajdusek and Gibbs succeeded in producing kuru in chimpanzees by inoculating infected human tissue.[33] Thus kuru became the first dementia in man demonstrated to be a virus-induced slow infection with an incubation period measured in years and with a progressive, accumulative pathology leading to death.

Another progressive human dementia known as Creutzfeldt-Jakob disease (CJD) has subsequently also been shown to be due to a slow virus infection.[34,35] Chimpanzees developed CJD 11 to 14 months following intracerebral inoculation of brain tissues from affected patients. Examination of the brains of infected animals once again reveals pathological changes similar to those found in kuru, including senile plaques.[36] Interestingly, as with kuru, material from infected organs appears to be capable of passing from CJD victims to susceptible people. One of the rare cases of this illness appears to have occurred as a result of a corneal transplant procedure in which the donor and the recipient both died of this dementing illness.[37] Another bizarre case occurred in a neurosurgeon who presumably became infected in the course of his work.[35]

In 1976 Daniel C. Gajdusek received the Nobel Prize in physiology and medicine in recognition of his important pioneering work in demonstrating that diseases such as kuru and CJD are largely infectious in origin and that the infections are due to these new kinds of infectious agents called slow viruses. In his Nobel Prize acceptance speech, Gajdusek also proposed a new name for these dementias caused by viruses, "transmissible virus dementia" (TVD). Might these TVDs in some way be responsible for Alzheimer's type senile dementia? Gajdusek and his colleague Clarence J. Gibbs, Jr., at the National Institute of Neurological and Communicative Disorders and Stroke of the National Institutes of Health at Bethesda, Maryland, have already begun to accumulate cases in which they believe they have been successful in transmitting the human Alzheimer's type dementias into animals.[38]

For example, a nurse's aide whom we'll call Helen had a father who had died at age 63 of a progressive dementia. Helen also had a sister, approximately her own age, who was hospitalized for psychiatric illness. Helen was married and had worked as a nurse's aide for 10 years when, at age 51, she began to have memory problems. She found she couldn't concentrate and she was unable to carry out her routine chores at home. She began to get lost. Also she began to have difficulty handling a knife and fork. She complained of headaches on her left side. Five months after the appearance of the first symptom, Helen's husband observed that she couldn't think of the proper word when she wanted to say something and that she put her clothing on backwards. A psychiatrist interviewed Helen and noted that she tended to ramble from topic to topic when she spoke, had difficulty speaking, and had a flat affect (inappropriately blunted emotional responses). Three months after this psychiatric interview, the patient was unaware of her location and was unable to perform simple arithmetic. At this point, eight months after the onset of Helen's condition, an extensive neurological workup was performed. Radioactively labeled air was injected into the fluid which surrounds the brain and spinal cord in order to provide a picture of the outline of the brain tissue. It revealed an increase in the fluid cavities of the brain and degeneration of the cortex, or outer layer, of the brain. Nine months after the first symptoms had developed, an operation was performed in which a small hole was drilled through Helen's skull. A piece of brain tissue was removed from the area below Helen's left temple. Pathologists examined the tissue and found neurofibrillary tangles and senile plaques. A diagnosis of Alzheimer's disease of early onset was made on the basis of these findings.

Gibbs and Gajdusek then took the brain tissue which had been removed from Helen's brain by the neurosurgeons. They put the tissue into a solution and injected the tissue suspension into the brains and into the blood vessels of different species of monkeys. Twenty-seven months after the injections, a spider monkey began to develop signs of a neurological illness. About 30 months after injection, a squirrel monkey developed neurological signs, and the same occurred in a capuchin monkey 40 months after the injections. These monkeys went on to develop a neurological illness which was indistinguishable from kuru and CJD! Examination of the brains of these monkeys revealed findings essentially identical to those in monkeys with kuru or CJD. This included the presence of senile plaques. Tangles, as always, were not observed in the brains of animals with the illness.

Helen was still reported to be living 10 years following the onset of her illness. Her illness has continued and has progressed slowly over the years.

Another woman, whom we'll call Barbara, also had a family history of dementia. However, the illness was even more manifest in Barbara's family than in Helen's. Barbara's father died of dementia at age 54. A brother died of progressive dementia after experiencing convulsions. Her brother's brain was examined at autopsy and revealed numerous neurofibrillary tangles and senile plaques, the hallmarks of Alzheimer's disease. A sister of Barbara's has also begun to show signs of dementia.

Barbara had been an excellent student in high school and college.

At 42 she began to have difficulty doing her housework. She also was noticed repeating things which she had just said. Three years later she was severely demented. When asked the names of common objects, she misnamed them. The following year she was admitted to a state psychiatric hospital because of her condition. In the hospital she developed uncontrollable jerking movements of her arms. She also developed convulsions. Her muscles became spastic and rigid. Almost six years after she began repeating things she had just said, she died.

An autopsy revealed a brain which had decayed and had shrunken in size. The characteristic features of Alzheimer's disease were present in the brain. PHFs 800 Å in length were seen by use of an electron microscope. The tangles were spread throughout the cortex and were particularly dense in the temporal region and the hippocampus. Material from the autopsied organs was injected into several kinds of monkeys and other primates. A squirrel monkey developed a neurological illness resulting in death a short time following observation of the condition. The monkey's brain had been injected with material from Barbara's brain approximately two years before the monkey developed the fatal condition. The squirrel monkey's brain revealed pathological changes which *did not* include neurofibrillary tangles or senile plaques. Furthermore, the researchers were successful in reproducing the squirrel monkey's condition by further inoculations of the monkey's brain substance in fellow primates of his own species as well as others.

What do these exciting findings tell us about Alzheimer's disease? Is it really one of these strange, newly discovered viral conditions which incubates for years and then suddenly begins to express itself and slowly, insidiously kills the host? If it is a virus, then how is it spread? Why does it run in families, at least in certain cases? Can we develop a vaccine against it?

The puzzle is really quite intricate, and these landmark findings of Gajdusek and Gibbs are only small parts of a much larger mosaic which will provide the answers to all of the above questions. Many of the other pieces of the puzzle have been found, and their contour and approximate location within the broader matrix will be described in the following pages. Other essential pieces are still entirely missing. But what is the significance of the observations described above?

It does appear that at least some forms of senility and specifically of Alzheimer's senility could possibly be caused by, or activated by, a virus. The virus may be a slow virus, closely related to that causing kuru and CJD in man and scrapie and mink encephalopathy in animals. Thus far, only the two cases of Helen and Barbara described above appear to have been shown to have been transmissible. The transmissible agent could have been a virus. In both of those cases there was a very strong familial (genetic) factor predisposing toward the development of the condition.

It is entirely possible that Alzheimer's disease, in common with innumerable other medical conditions such as high blood pressure, psychosis, and dementia itself, is a syndrome, or final common pathway, with many different possible causes. Viral factors could be important in the causation of at least some cases of the familial, early-onset type of Alzheimer's disease.

If it is a virus, at least in certain instances, can we, in these instances, prevent it, treat it, arrest it, or kill it? "It is in the power of man to make parasitic maladies disappear from the face of the globe." So stated the great Louis Pasteur more than a century ago.[39] Nevertheless, one hundred and ten years later mankind is on the verge of declaring total victory in wiping out one, and only one, parasitic malady from the planet. Even this singular victory, over smallpox, remains tenuous and, tragically, may ultimately prove temporary. In order to be certain of victory, mankind feels obligated to preserve specimens of the virus in at least a few laboratories around the world, for identification purposes. The last smallpox outbreak originated from one of these "archival" laboratories in England. Furthermore, with the discontinuation of universal vaccination and natural immune factors, the peoples of the earth will be extremely sensitive to any reoccurrence of the dread disease.

For the slow viruses, host immune factors have not been identified as yet. No measures are known at present which can halt or even retard the inexorable progress of these conditions. Nevertheless, Pasteur's bold statement certainly remains a modern hope.

To return to our unraveling of the mysteries of senility and Alzheimer's disease, the experiments of Gadjusek and Gibbs do seem to bring us to some other interesting conclusions. It will be recalled that PHFs have been found only in human beings. Senile plaques do not seem to be species-specific. Nevertheless, when Barbara's condition was transferred to monkeys, these animals developed neurological illnesses without either of these pathological manifestations. There was rather the pathological picture of a "spongiform encephalopathy." Another way of saying this is to say that the brain was decayed and filled with "holes," much like a sponge. Neither plaques nor tangles were present. It would appear that the plaques and tangles are unique scars of illness. Certainly they are not the illness itself. Tangles seem to be a uniquely human form of scarification. Plaques seem to be more general. Certainly in animals the causative illness can occur without either of these manifestations. Perhaps the same is true in people. This would help to explain why cases of senile dementia are encountered in which persons show one or another of these hallmarks in the absence of the other.

We have already said that the occurrence of senile plaques increases as progressively older populations are examined. We also have shown that, unlike neurofibrillary tangles, senile plaques are to be found in various species of animals, at least in association with certain disease processes. Are there animals in which the incidence of senile plaque formation in the brain increases with aging? In other words, are senile plaques a uniquely human aging phenomenon or a more general one?

The answer appears to be that in at least one other, rather distantly related mammal, the dog, senile plaques have been observed accompanying the aging process. This observation was first reported in 1956.[40] It has since been shown that the plaques in the aged dog may closely mimic those of humans. Some of the plaques consist of an amyloid core surrounded by neuronal processes and reactive cells.[41,42] No neurofibrillary tangles are found. However, the brains of aging dogs with these senile plaques show decay very similar to the decay often seen in human brains with senile plaques. That is, the frontal and temporal outer portions of the brain decay, and a corresponding deepening of the sulci, or "grooves," of the brains of dogs, as of humans, is often found.

Hence the dog may be an excellent model for the study of human senility. But are these brain changes truly "senile changes" in the behavioral sense of the word? Do dogs, or other animals, become forgetful and, ultimately, demented the way humans sometimes do?

The answer to this question, while crucial, is largely unavailable at this time. In one study, old monkeys mastered a set of problems as efficiently as middle-aged monkeys, but the middle-aged monkeys retained more of what they had learned 24 hours later.[43] Raymond Bartus, a behavioral scientist, has conducted a series of investigations of the memory abilities of rhesus monkeys.[44,45] When he compares the performance of young monkeys with that of aged monkeys, he finds that the aged monkeys do considerably worse on tasks which require monkeys to learn a new behavior and to demonstrate knowledge of that new behavior a short while later. He describes his aged rhesus monkeys as being inferior to young monkeys in "short-term memory." This "short-term memory deficit" is also the first sign of Alzheimer's disease in people. Also, many aged humans display a loss of short-term memory abilities. Indeed, a decrease in short-term memory is the earliest manifestation of so-called "benign senescent forgetfulness."

These are interesting findings, but what about brain changes and senility in animals? We have shown that in humans the brain changes seen in Alzheimer's disease have been associated with a decrease in thinking capacity. No such association has yet been made in animal studies.[46] Hence we are faced with the possibility that not only the characteristic Alzheimer's neurofibrillary tangles but also the progressive dementia with which they are associated are distinctly human phenomena.

The third characteristic pathological change in the brains of patients with Alzheimer's disease is "granulovacuolar degeneration." This is really a descriptive term for certain changes which appear inside cells. Specifically, the interior of a cell undergoing this form of degeneration becomes crowded with fluid-filled "vacuoles" as well as with granular material. Granulovacuolar degeneration is found to some extent in the hippocampal area of the brains of a majority of elderly persons.[47] An increased concentration of granulovacuolar degeneration in certain areas of the hippocampus is very significantly related to the clinical finding of dementia. Ninety percent of persons with more than 90 percent of hippocampal neurons undergoing granulovacuolar degeneration are seriously demented. Almost all of these persons will be found to have large numbers of senile plaques and neurofibrillary tangles.[17]

We have seen that modern pathological studies have demonstrated conclusively that what was formerly known as "Alzheimer's presenile dementia" and is now known simply as "Alzheimer's disease" is the major cause of senility in man. Alzheimer's disease is marked by decay of the frontotemporal and cortical areas of the brain. It is also characterized by certain distinctive, but not necessarily unique, pathological findings. These findings are neurofibrillary tangles, senile plaques, and granulovacuolar degeneration. Each of these pathological hallmarks, individually, is positively associated with progressive idiopathic (senile) dementia in man. Each of these pathologic hall-marks is also seen increasingly frequently in many nondemented aged individuals.

The hippocampus appears to be the primary portion of the brain with Alzheimer's type pathological changes. The hippocampus is also the primary anatomic locus of short-term memory. Short-term memory loss is the earliest sign of senile dementia and of memory loss associated with aging. Hence the frequently observed tendency for elderly persons to forget the names of people to whom they are in-troduced and to forget where they have placed objects may be a behavioral expression of the progressive, bilateral, Alzheimer's type changes in the hippocampus. This hypothesis is, of course, potentially testable. Scientists could identify a group of persons with and without short-term memory impairment and, after the demise of the in-dividuals concerned, examine the brains for evidence of pathological change in the hippocampus and elsewhere. Theoretically, this is not a particularly difficult experiment. Logistically, however, the barriers preventing such a study—examining elderly persons for short-term memory impairment shortly before their demise; ensuring that they do not suffer from an illness other than Alzheimer's disease which can itself interfere with cognition; obtaining permission from the family to perform an autopsy, etc.—are formidable.

The amygdala and the entire cerebral cortex, concerned with emo-tional and cognitive functioning respectively, are also involved in the later stages of Alzheimer's disease. The involvement of these brain structures may explain not only the widespread thinking disturbances accompanying senile dementia but also many of the emotional distur-bances which occur in the moderate and late stage of the illness.

Senile plaques are known to occur in some mammals in association with age-related changes and also in association with viral and specifically "slow virus" disease. Some animals have also been shown to have short-term memory loss in association with aging. No mam-mals other than man have been shown to have the characteristic neurofibrillary tangles known as PHFs. No animals other than man have been shown to undergo the behavioral changes which we associate with senile dementia.

An analysis of these facts does seem to give us important clues to the origins of senile dementia in man. The human condition does ap-pear to be, in some ways, unique. However, similar kinds of condi-tions, which do not express themselves in precisely the same fashion, do appear to occur in other animals. Together, the human and the infrahuman conditions seem to indicate an interactive process between aging and viruses that results in age-related cognitive decline and dementia. Evidence has accumulated for a possible viral role in senile dementia. Certainly, virus-like agents can cause dementias resembling, but not identical to, Alzheimer's disease. One laboratory appears to have transmitted two cases of familial Alzheimer's disease by inoculation into animals. This work will have to be replicated in other centers before its true significance can be assessed.

We now know something about the structural changes observed in the brains of persons with Alzheimer's dementia. Structural changes do not exist in a vacuum. What are the chemical changes? What physiological changes occur? We have implicated slow viruses and alluded to familial factors in Alzheimer's disease. What exactly are the supposed origins of this commonly seen, but so little known, malady?

Notes

1. Robbins, S. L., *Pathology,* 3d ed., W. B. Saunders Company, Philadelphia, 1967, p. 573.
2. Rennie, E., and Hollenberg, N. K., Cardiomythology and marathons. *New England J. Med.* 301: 103–104, 1979.
3. Currens, J. H., and White, P. D., Half a century of running: Clinical, physiologic and autopsy findings in the case of Clarence De Mar ("Mr. Marathon"). *New England J. Med.* 265: 988–993, 1961.
4. Bassler, T. J., Marathon running and immunity to atherosclerosis. *Ann. NY Acad. Sci.* 301: 579–592, 1977.
5. Bassler, T. J., and Cardello, F. P., Fiber-feeding and atherosclerosis. *JAMA* 235: 1841–1842, 1976.
6. Noakes, T. D., Opie, L. H., Rose, A. G., and Kleynhaus, P. H. T., Autopsy-proved coronary atherosclerosis in marathon runners. *New England J. Med.* 301:86–89, 1979.
7. Corsellis, J. A. N., and Evans, P. H., The relation of stenosis of the extracranial cerebral arteries to mental disorder and cerebral degeneration in old age, *Proc. Vth Int. Congr. Neuropath.,* 1965, p. 546.
8. Worm-Petersen, J., and Pakkenberg, H., "Atherosclerosis of cerebral arteries, pathological and clinical correlations," *J. Geront.* 23: 445, 1968.
9. Roth, M., Tomlinson, B. E., and Blessed, G., Correlation between scores for dementia and counts of "senile plaques" in cerebral grey matter of elderly subjects. *Nature* 209: 109, 1966.
10. Blessed, G., Tomlinson, B. E., and Roth, M., The association between quantitative measures of dementia and of senile changes in the cerebral grey matter of elderly subjects. *Brit. J. Psychiat.* 114: 797–811, 1968.

11. Tomlinson, B. E., Blessed, G., and Roth, M., Observations on the brains of non-demented old people. *J. Neurol. Sci.* 7: 331-356, 1968.
12. Tomlinson, B. E., Blessed, G., and Roth, M., Observations on the brains of demented old people. *J. Neurol. Sci.* 11: 205-242, 1970.
13. Hachinski, V. C., Lassen, N. A., and Marshall, J., Multi-infarct dementia: A cause of mental deterioration in the elderly. *Lancet,* July 27, 1974, pp. 207-209.
14. Alzheimer, A., Uber eine eigenartige Erkrankung der Hirnrinde. *Centralblatt Nervenheilk. Psychiat.* 18: 177, 1907.
15. Kidd, M., Alzheimer's disease—an electron microsurgical study. *Brain* 87: 307-320, 1964.
16. Terry, R. D., Gonotas, N. K., and Weiss, M., Ultrastructural studies in Alzheimer's presenile dementia. *Amer. J. Path.* 44: 269-297, 1964.
17. Tomlinson, B. E., and Henderson, G., Some quantitative cerebral findings in normal and demented old people. In *Neurobiology of Aging,* ed. by Robert D. Terry and Samuel Gershon, Raven Press, New York, 1976, pp. 183-204.
18. Martland, H. S., Punch drunk. *JAMA* 91: 1103-1107, 1928.
19. Wisniewski, H. M., Ghetti, B., and Terry, R. D., Neuritis (senile) plaques and filamentous changes in aged rhesus monkeys. *J. Neuropath. Exp. Neurol.* 32: 566-584, 1973.
20. Papez, J. W., A proposed mechanism of emotion. *Arch. Neurol. Psychiat.,* 38: 725, 1937.
21. Rosvold, H. E., Mirsky, A. F., and Pribram, K. H., Influence of amygdalectomy on social behavior in monkeys. *Comp. Physiol. Psychol.* 47: 173, 1954.
22. Ganong, W. F., *Review of Medical Physiology,* Lange, Los Altos, Calif., 1971.
23. Itil, T. M., and Reisberg, B., Pharmacologic treatment of aggressive syndromes. In *Current Psychiatric Therapies,* Vol. 18, ed. by Jules H. Masserman, Grune & Stratton, Inc., 1979, pp. 137-142.
24. Hornykiewicz, O., Dopamine (3-hydroxytyramine) and brain function. *Pharmacol. Rev.* 18: 925, 1966.
25. Glenner, G. G., Ein, D., and Terry, W. D., The immunoglobulin origin of amyloid. *Amer. J. Med.* 52: 141-147, 1972.
26. Glenner, G. G., Terry, W. D., and Isersky, C., Amyloidosis: Its nature and pathogenesis. *Sem. Hematol.* 10: 65-86, 1973.
27. Klatzo, I., Gajdusek, D. C., and Zigas, V., Pathology of kuru. *Lab. Invest.* 8: 799-847, 1959.
28. Besnoit, C., La tremblante ou névrite péripherique enzootique du mouton. *Rev. Vit. Toulouse* 24: 265-277, 333-343, 1899.
29. Gibbs, C. J., Jr., Search for infectious etiology in chronic and subacute degenerative diseases of the central nervous system. *Curr. Topics Microbiol. Immunol.* 40: 44-58, 1967.

30. Chandler, R. L., Encephalopathy in mice produced by innoculation with scrapie brain material. *Lancet* 1: 1378–1379, 1961.
31. Wisniewski, H. M., Bruce, M. E., and Fraser, H., Infectious aetiology of neuritic (senile) plaques in mice. *Science* 190: 1108–1110, 1975.
32. Fraser, H., and Bruce, M. E., Argyrophilic plaques in mice innoculated with scrapie from particular sources. *Lancet* 1: 617, 1973.
33. Gajdusek, D. C., and Gibbs, J. C., Jr., Slow, latent, and temperate virus infections of the central nervous system. *Res. Publ. Assoc. Rev. Nerv. Ment. Dis.* 44: 254–280, 1968.
34. Gajdusek, D. C., Unconventional viruses and the origin and disappearance of kuru. In *Les Prix Nobel,* Nobel Foundation, Stockholm, 1977, pp. 167–216.
35. Traub, R., Gajdusek, D. C., and Gibbs, C. J., Jr., Transmissible virus dementia: The relations of transmissible spongiform encephalopathy to Creutzfeldt-Jakob disease. In *Aging and Dementia,* ed. by M. Kinsbourne and L. Smith, Spectrum, New York, 1977, pp. 91–172.
36. Chou, S. M., and Martin, J. D., Kuru plaques in a case of Creutzfeldt-Jakob disease. *Acta Neuropath.* (Berlin) 17: 150–155, 1971.
37. Duffy, P., Wolf, J., Collins, G., DeVoe, A. G., Strecten, B., and Cowen, D., Possible person-to-person transmission of Creutzfeldt-Jakob disease. *New England J. Med.* 299: 692–693, 1974.
38. Gibbs, C. J., Jr., and Gajdusek, D. C., Subacute spongiform virus encephalopathies: The transmissible virus dementias. In *Alzheimer's Disease: Senile Dementia and Related Disorders (Aging,* Vol. 7), ed. by R. Katzman, R. D. Terry, and K. L. Bick, Raven Press, New York, 1978, pp. 559–575.
39. De Kruif, Paul, *Microbe Hunters,* Harcourt, Brace and Company, New York, 1926, p. 97.
40. Braunmuhl, A., Kongophile Angiopathie und senile Plaques bei greisen Hunden. *Arch. Psychiat. Nervenker.* 194: 396–414, 1956.
41. Wisniewski, H. M., and Terry, R. D., Re-examination of the pathogenesis of the senile plaque. In *Progress in Neuropathology,* Vol. 11, ed. by H. M. Zimmerman, Grune & Stratton, New York, 1973, pp. 1–26.
42. Wisniewski, H., Johnson, A. B., Raine, C. S., Kay, M. J., and Terry, R. D., Senile plaques and cerebral amyloidosis in aged dogs: A histochemical study. *Lab. Invest.* 23: 287–296, 1970.
43. Medin, D. L., O'Neil, P., Smeltz, E., and Davis, R. T., Age differences in retention of concurrent discrimination problems in monkeys. *J. Geront.* 28: 63–67, 1973.
44. Bartus, R. T., Fleming, D. L., and Johnson, H. R., The effects of aging on primate short-term memory, sensory processing and learning. *Neuroscience Abstr.* 3: 714, 1977.
45. Bartus, R. T., Fleming, D. L., and Johnson, H. R., Aging in the rhesus

monkey: debilitating effects on short-term memory. *J. Geront.* 3(6): 858, 1978.

46. Brizzee, K. R., Ordy, J. M., Hofer, H., and Kaak, B., Animal models for the study of senile brain disease and aging changes in the brain. In *Alzheimer's Disease: Senile Dementia and Related Disorders (Aging,* Vol. 7), ed. by R. Katzman, R. D. Terry, and K. L. Bick, Raven Press, New York, 1978, pp. 515–554.

47. Tomlinson, B. E., and Kitchener, D., Granulovacuolar degeneration of the hippocampus pyramidal cells. *J. Path.* 106: 165–185, 1972.

Chapter 3

Origins of Alzheimer's Disease

WE HAVE SEEN THAT Alzheimer's disease accounts for the majority of cases of senile dementia. We have also found that Alzheimer's disease causes characteristic changes in the structure of the brain and that some of these changes, such as decay, are visible to the unaided eye, whereas others, such as plaques and tangles, can be seen under a microscope. What are the effects of Alzheimer's disease on the chemistry and the functioning of the brain? Can these chemical and functional changes tell us more about the origins of the deficits found in senility and perhaps give us clues regarding the treatment of senility?

We do not yet understand exactly how the brain works, but we do know much more about its workings than we once did. We know that the brain contains nerve cells, or "neurons," which are central to thought, emotion, and behavior. These neurons in some way carry out all of the "higher" activities of the brain. The other cells of the brain appear to exist solely for the support and nourishment of the neurons. Neurons are unique in the ways in which they can communicate with each other. We have learned that they do not communicate directly—they never touch each other—but by chemicals. When a neuron "wants" to communicate with another neuron, it sends out a chemical. The other neuron is specially adapted so that it can receive this chemical message. These adaptations are called "receptors."

Every neuron is specialized so that it secretes (transmits) only one particular kind of chemical messenger. It either secretes its chemical messenger or it does not; i.e., it either sends out a message or it doesn't. The brain contains merely a handful of important chemical messengers. One of these messengers is a substance known as "acetylcholine."

Neurons, of course, exist not only in the brain but all over the body. Wherever neurons are found, they communicate with each other using these special chemicals, which are appropriately known as "neurotransmitters." In the human body, whenever we decide to move a muscle, a neuron secretes acetylcholine, telling the muscle to contract. Hence we say that acetylcholine is the neurotransmitter substance used to communicate messages for voluntary muscles to contract. Acetylcholine is the neurotransmitter for voluntary muscle contraction whether we want to blink an eye or move a toe.

The brain, of course, is even more complex. We have not yet reached the level of knowledge whereby we can say that a particular neurotransmitter produces a specific brain activity. For example, we do not know which neurotransmitter is responsible for short-term memory. We do know, however, that particular brain cells secrete specific neurotransmitter substances. We also know that acetylcholine is one of the major substances (others are dopamine, serotonin, and noradrenalin).

To return to our examination of the brains of persons with Alzheimer's disease, if one examines advanced cases of persons with Alzheimer's dementia after death, at the time when they come to autopsy, one finds, as we have said, decay. If one examines the brains of elderly persons without Alzheimer's disease, there is usually no decay. Upon closer examination the decay in Alzheimer's brains is seen to be centered in the temporal lobes. It is roughly symmetrical; i.e., it appears roughly the same on both sides of the head. Cortical areas outside the temporal lobes decay to a much lesser extent, and other areas of the brain show no decay at all.

If one examines brain material from the temporal lobes of persons with Alzheimer's disease (decayed or not) one comes up with some startling findings. First of all, one finds that only the neurons decay. There is no loss of the supportive cells known as the glia. This contrasts with findings in normal subjects the same age, in whom there is ordinarily preservation of neurons and loss of glia. All right, then, whatever this disease is, it is destroying the nerve cells of the cortex, especially in the temporal lobe, and leaving scars (plaques and tangles). Which nerve cells does it destroy?

The neurotransmitters are manufactured in the neurons which secrete them. Enzymes catalyze the chemical reactions which result in the neurotransmitter production. The more active the cell is in producing neurotransmitter substance, the greater will be the quantity of the enzymes responsible for their synthesis. For most cellular reactions, one enzyme is found to be most important for the reaction to occur. That enzyme is known as the "rate-limiting enzyme."

The rate-limiting enzyme for the synthesis of acetylcholine is known as "choline acetyl transferase," or "CAT" for short. CAT activity can be measured in a quantity of brain substance. The amount of CAT activity tells us to what extent the cells in that portion of the brain are able to manufacture acetylcholine.

When we measure the CAT activity in the temporal lobes of the brains of persons with Alzheimer's disease and compare it with that in normal persons the same age, we find that in Alzheimer's patients CAT activity is only 35 to 40 percent of what it should be. Furthermore, the reduction in CAT activity in Alzheimer's disease is twice as much as the loss of nerve cells from the whole temporal lobe. Hence there appears to be selective destruction of the neurons which secrete acetylcholine (the cholinergic neurons) in the temporal lobes of persons with Alzheimer's disease.[1]

This is indeed interesting. Alzheimer's disease selectively destroys the neurons secreting acetylcholine. Does it attack any of the other neurons in the temporal lobes?

To a lesser extent, it appears that it does. Indeed, in one way or another it appears to affect all of the major neurotransmitters of the temporal lobe of the cortex. Noradrenalin-secreting neurons are also reduced in Alzheimer's patients.[2,3] Receptor chemical binding studies have shown that the receptors for acetylcholine and noradrenalin apparently remain intact in the diseased portions of the Alzheimer's brains. However, receptors for other neurotransmitter systems apparently are altered.

If cholinergic neurons are selectively destroyed in the brains of persons with Alzheimer's disease, does this explain some of the behavior changes seen in senility?

It appears that it does have some effect on behavior. We can block the cholinergic system chemically using drugs known as "anticholinergics." Some anticholinergic drugs are well known. An example is curare, the South American Indian arrow poison which blocks acetylcholine transmission to the muscles, resulting in paralysis. Another is belladonna (bella = beautiful, donna = lady) from the deadly nightshade plant. Formerly it was fashionable for women to drop belladonna on their eyes. The anticholinergic effect would cause their pupils to dilate, making the ladies more attractive. It has been known for many years that if one gives belladonna or similar anticholinergic drugs which are capable of entering the brain, amnesia results.[4] More recently, Drachman and Leavitt gave scopolamine (a belladonna derivative) to young adult volunteers. They found memory effects very similar to those which occur in senile dementia.[5]

The relationship between acetylcholine and memory and learning does not appear to be a simple one. On the basis of the most recent experiments, notably those of Ken Davis and his associates, we believe that either too much or too little acetylcholine in the brain may interfere with memory and learning.[6] Even the more severe behavioral changes observed in the final stages of Alzheimer's disease can be largely explained on the basis of changes in the acetylcholine content of the brain. We know that substances which produce either too much or too little acetylcholine are capable of causing hallucinations and severe thinking disturbances, in other words, psychosis.

If these cholinergic and to a lesser extent the other neurotransmitter systems are being selectively destroyed by Alzheimer's disease, is there anything which we can do about it? Can we replace these chemical messengers? If we can replace them, will it do any good, particularly since the neurons are being destroyed anyway?

Apparently we can increase the quantities of these neurotransmitters in the brain. In fact, we may be able to increase the acetylcholine in the brain simply by eating the proper foods! Furthermore, these "replacement" chemicals may reduce the severity of the disease! We will have more to say on this in the chapter on treatments. But first of all, what are the other fundamental changes of Alzheimer's disease? If we understood these other basic changes, perhaps we could treat them as well.

One of the very important physiological changes which is found in the brains of Alzheimer's patients is in the flow of blood to the brain. As mentioned earlier, modern techniques have been developed which enable scientists to determine not only how much blood is going to the brain but also to which parts of the brain the blood travels.

The most modern procedure employs a radioactive labeled inert gas, xenon 133. In this procedure a cap surrounded by geiger counters is placed over a person's head so that the radioactive gas can be precisely located in the different brain regions. The xenon 133 isotope is then mixed with ordinary air and inhaled.* It enters the lungs and is absorbed into the bloodstream. In the blood it goes to the heart and then to the entire body. When the isotope travels through the brain, its presence is detected by the geiger counters. Since the concentration of the isotope is the same throughout the bloodstream, the quantity of radiation in any region of the brain will depend upon how much blood is flowing through the region. The more radiation found in a brain region, the more blood must be flowing to that region. Naturally, computers are employed to analyze the information obtained by the many geiger counters located above every area of the head. The result is a picture which can show us the regions of the brain to which the blood is being shunted.

These procedures have demonstrated that there is a definite overall decrease in the amount of blood going to the brain in persons with senile dementia. Furthermore, the more severe the degree of intellectual deficit, the less blood flowing to the brain.[7,8,9]

Studies have been conducted in which the blood flow to the brain was measured prior to the demise of demented individuals. After their death the brains of these persons were examined. The areas in which the blood flow to the brain was decreased were the same areas in which the brain decay and pathological changes of Alzheimer's disease were found![10] Hence the changes in the blood flow to the brain seem to provide scientists with a yardstick for measuring, during life, Alzheimer's brain changes which ordinarily can only be observed directly on the brains of deceased persons.

There are other ways in which cerebral blood flow changes seem to reflect actual brain changes classically found only at autopsy. For example, we mentioned earlier that neurons are the brain tissues which tend to decay in Alzheimer's disease. The neuronal cell bodies are located mainly in parts of the brain known as "gray matter." We can examine the blood flow to the gray matter of Alzheimer's patients and compare it with the proportion of blood which goes to the gray matter

---

* Formerly, the Scandinavian scientists who pioneered this technique had to inject the xenon isotope into the carotid artery in the neck. Fortunately, this is no longer necessary and the radioactive gas can be inhaled directly. There are no needles or injections, and the only discomfort for the subject is in being asked to sit quietly and not move around too much, which is occasionally difficult for a senile patient.

of younger, healthy persons. Investigators have done this, and indeed they have discovered that both the overall amount of gray matter and the percentage of blood going to the gray matter are decreased in the Alzheimer's patients.[10,11]

Not only do cerebral blood flow studies appear to give us information on the pathological changes occurring in the brain and the overall degree of dementia; they also appear to relate to the specific kinds of problems experienced by senile persons. For example, we know that the brain is divided into two halves, a left hemisphere and a right hemisphere. In the majority of persons who are right-handed, the left half of the brain is primarily responsible for speech and verbal abilities in general. Studies conducted with senile persons have found that only when blood flow is observed to be decreased to the speech centers on the left side of the brain does the impaired person display significant deficits in verbal abilities.[12]

Other kinds of dynamic relationships between blood flow and deficits have already been found. Demented persons appear to lose the ability to "activate," or increase, the blood flow to areas of the brain in which cognitive ability is impaired. For instance, if an unimpaired person is asked to do calculations, blood flow to the right side of the brain ordinarily will increase. However, a demented or impaired person who already has less blood flow to this portion of the right side of the brain also may show less ability to increase the blood flow when required to perform the calculations.

We have seen that blood flow changes relate to the pathological findings and the clinical findings known to occur in senility. Do these changes have anything to do with the loss of cholinergic neurons described in the opening pages of this chapter? The answer is "perhaps." We know that physiologically less blood flow to certain areas of the brain translates into less oxygen reaching these brain regions. According to John Blass of the New York Hospital–Cornell Medical Center, "The synthesis of acetylcholine from labelled precursors is exquisitely sensitive to hypoxia.* Hippocampal acetylcholine may be particularly sensitive."[13] These speculations are supported by the recent findings that hypoxia produced deficits in short-term memory in mice very similar to those seen in people with Alzheimer's disease.[14]

Hence the observed changes in cholinergic neurons may be the

* "Hypoxia" means "decreased oxygen availability."

result of the changes in blood flow and resulting hypoxia rather than the other way around. Until the proper experiments are designed and carried out, this will remain a "chicken and the egg" conundrum. However, we can treat the blood flow changes by giving substances which tend to increase the flow of blood and the metabolism of the brain. These treatments remain the most popular and the most successful current pharmacological approaches to Alzheimer's disease. Again, we shall have more to say about these later. For now, let's return to our quest for the origins of the condition. We have seen how biochemical (neurotransmitter), physiological (blood flow), and structural (pathological) changes all occur and have explored their interrelationships in Alzheimer's dementia. However, if we are to understand the cause of this enormous health problem, we must dig deeper. We must get to the fundamental biological mechanisms of the disease.

Inevitably we come to chromosomes. These, of course, are the fundamental, genetic coders of life. They contain the information which, together with certain environmental influences, makes us what we are. Throughout our lifetimes, in each individual cell, chromosomes manufacture RNA, which in turn provides the template for the synthesis of proteins. The latter are the biological substrate for much of cellular structure and function. This chromosome—RNA—protein interaction appears to be responsible in part for cellular differentiation, that is, for the process which makes some cells nerve cells and others blood cells, etc. It may also be related to the pathological process which occasionally causes cells to become malignant.

We do not know the secret of aging. Scientists can only speculate on the causes of the process which makes all organisms age and die. Certainly death is "programmed." In other words, it must be built into the genetic material of the cell. One plausible theory of aging in general is that it results from the progressive accumulation of genetic "errors" which accrue from the breakage and damage to which chromosomes are subjected over the course of a lifetime. These genetic errors would be expressed as deficient protein and enzyme manufacture by the cells, which in turn would decrease their ability to function in any number of ways. One important area in which a cellular genetic error may be crucial to the life of a cell is in the immune system. This, in its least complicated form, is the process by which cells, and the body in general, respond to foreign "antigens"—usually proteins—by the manufacture of antibodies. This delicate system is undoubtedly dependent upon the competence of the chromosomal-RNA-protein system to recognize new antigenic material and to respond to it rapidly and accurately by the manufacture of exactly the right antibody. If this system becomes impaired in any way, then the organism becomes more susceptible to disease and may succumb earlier.

However, we know that in the case of modern man, it is not infectious or parasitic disease which often causes old age and death. Rather, it is processes such as arthritis, in which the joints and tissues seem to decay; heart disease, in which cardiac functioning is compromised; cancer; and brain failure. The immune system would seem to have little to do with these important causes of aging and death in man.

Not true.

One aspect of the immune system, as we have said, is that the body manufactures antibodies to foreign antigens. To do this, the body must be capable of distinguishing between its own material and foreign material. In recent years scientists have discovered that one way in which the immune system may malfunction is in the body's manufacturing antibodies against its own antigenic substance. In other words, the body actually makes substances which can destroy it. This new kind of disease has been appropriately termed an ''autoimmune disease.''

Scientists now know of many different kinds of autoimmune diseases. The most important one for this discussion is rheumatoid arthritis. In this generalized disease, strongly associated with aging, the joints become narrowed and twisted, nodules develop, and overall bodily functioning is markedly impaired. All of this appears to be the result of the body's manufacture of substances to destroy itself—in other words, immune incompetence.

Cancer also may be related to the chromosomal and immune systems. Clearly, cancer results when the genetic instructions with which cells regulate their growth and development under normal circumstances go awry. It seems that many different kinds of processes and events can cause this to occur. A virus, in the case of certain cancers, enters a cell, attaches itself to the genetic material, and changes the cellular manufacturing process directly. In other cases chemical carcinogens—any one of thousands of different substances—interfere with the genetic code, and, when present in sufficiently large quantities, will cause particularly sensitive cellular lines to become cancerous. Radiation, which also interferes with genetic processes, sometimes results in cancer. Heredity also appears to play a role in a variety of ways. Genetic incompetence in certain cellular lines may be inherited directly, resulting in cancer of a particular tissue at a certain stage of life in all succeeding generations. Hereditary factors may also play an indirect role, making particular cellular genetic materials unusually sensitive to cancer-causing agents in the environment such as viruses and chemicals. Diet also seems to play some role in making cellular genetic material more or less sensitive to cancer-causing agents.

Hence cancer can be thought of as a biological "final common pathway" in which the genetic programming of a cellular line goes awry. Carcinogens are agents which promote this process by interfering with the cellular genome. Hence viruses, environmental chemicals, radiation, heredity factors, and dietary factors may all contribute, individually or in combination, to the fundamental genetic changes which result in cancer.

Alzheimer's disease appears to result from a very similar process. Evidence from many different sources indicates that the process is approximately as shown in Figure 3–1.

Processes which predispose to chromosomal breakage or coding

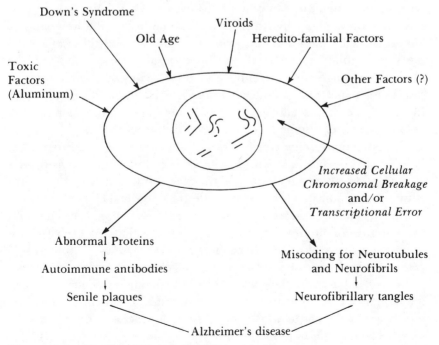

Figure 3.1 Possible Origins of Alzheimer's Disease

error, individually or in combination, predispose to the ultimate development of Alzheimer's disease. We're referring to specific and as yet unidentified kinds of chromosomal breaks and errors—namely, those genetic traumas which would result in an increase in autoimmune antibodies and/or miscoding for neurotubules and neurofibrils.

Initial evidence that cellular chromosomal damage may be related to the development of senile dementia has been available for several years. In 1968 Nielson in Denmark compared women hospitalized with senile dementia with women of comparable age who were mentally intact. He found that the dementia patients had a significantly higher frequency of chromosome loss than did the others.[15] Lissy Jarvik and her co-workers conducted similar investigations and came to the same conclusions.[16,17,18] They examined white blood cells of elderly persons ranging in age from 77 to 93 years. They found that in some elderly people the proportion of cells missing one or more chromosomes was very high. As many as one in four cells had at least one missing chromosome in some elderly people. However, the frequency of missing chromosomes was not related to chronological age as such in their sample. Rather, it was strongly related to impaired mental functioning. They found a relationship between the proportion of cells with an abnormal number of chromosomes and psychological test performance on a whole spectrum of tasks. The higher the frequency of abnormal cells, the lower the scores on tests such as those of vocabulary, the ability to recite digits forwards and backwards, and the ability to arrange and to complete pictures. The correlation between test performance and chromosome loss was in the predicted direction in all of the 15 psychological tests which they administered. The greater the chromosome loss, the worse the performance.

Investigations being concluded by the Geriatric Study Program at N.Y.U., in collaboration with Harlow K. Fischman and his associates at the Cell Genetics Laboratory of the New York State Psychiatric Institute, have indicated that more subtle chromosomal changes may occur in Alzheimer's disease. Chromosomes replicate during cell division by dividing longitudinally. The replicated portions of each chromosome appear early in cell division and are known as "chromatids." Hence each chromosome consists of two chromatids. In the normal process of cell division the chromatids separate and each goes to one of the daughter cells to form a new chromosome. Frequently, however, separation of the chromatids is not a smooth process. The chromatids may become twisted around each other, resulting in breakage and the exchange of genetic material between the "sister chromatids" during mitosis. Geneticists have logically named this process "sister chromatid exchange."

In examining white blood cells from patients with Alzheimer's disease and comparing them with cells from persons of similar age without memory impairment, we have found an increase in sister chromatid exchanges in the Alzheimer's patients.[19] We have also found some indication that the increase in sister chromatid exchange level is dependent on the gravity of the disease. If verified, these findings might indicate that a variety of cellular chromosomal changes predispose to the development of Alzheimer's disease.

Recent investigations of the nature and activity of the genetic material in the brain cells of Alzheimer's patients give further support for the theory of an acquired genetic deficit. Donald Crapper and Umberto De Boni in Toronto have found an alteration in chromatin conformation in Alzheimer's disease.[20] Both neurons and the glial supportive brain tissue showed a marked decrease in transcriptionally active chromatin in Alzheimer's patients as compared with other patients the same age or as compared with patients with other forms of dementia. Hence in Alzheimer's disease there may be a deficit in the production of RNA from the chromosomal material. This in turn would lead to the production of abnormal proteins. One of the abnormal proteins may result in neurofibrillary tangles in place of normal brain microtubules. Support for this hypothesis has come from studies which have shown an immunologic relationship between Alzheimer's paired helical filament protein and normal brain microtubulin.[21]

Other abnormal proteins are undoubtedly produced by the altered RNA which is coded for by the damaged chromosomes. These new proteins may be interpreted by the body as foreign substances. The body may therefore produce antibodies against these new proteins. In the short term this process may result in senile plaques as a result of the metabolic processing and digestion of the resulting antigen-antibody complexes. Over the long term the destruction of the body's own neural tissue by antibodies may explain the destruction of the nerve cells themselves and the gradual atrophy of the brain which occurs.

Once again, these theories have received some support from scientific studies. Kalidas Nandy of the Boston University Medical Center has found that antineuron antibodies formed in the sera of aging mice appeared to play an important role in the age-related loss of nerve cells.[22] Subsequently he studied the levels of brain-reactive antibodies in the sera of patients with Alzheimer's disease.[23] He found that the Alzheimer's patients did indeed have significantly higher levels of such antibodies than age-matched control subjects.

We have seen how chromosomal breakage in the cells of the brain can result in abnormal cellular microtubules which may become neurofibrillary tangles and result in Alzheimer's disease. We have also traced the mechanism whereby chromosomal breakage may result in altered proteins which may provoke the production of "auto-anti-bodies" against the body's own substance. We have seen how this autoimmune disease may become visible as senile plaques—digested antigen-antibody complexes—and as brain decay. Once again the end result is Alzheimer's disease. Let us now return to the more immediate causes of the disease—specifically, the processes which produce the genetic and chromosomal changes which set in motion the pathological developments described above.

The primary processes which trigger the sequence of events leading to Alzheimer's disease appear to be varied. They include (1) aging in general, (2) transmissible agents which we shall call "viroids," (3) hereditary and familial predispositions, (4) Down's syndrome, (5) environmental toxins such as aluminium, and other as yet undiscovered factors. Each of these primary etiologies contributes to the specific kinds of genetic changes which result in Alzheimer's type brain failure. Undoubtedly the most important is age itself.

The incidence of Alzheimer's disease increases from the time of its earliest appearance in middle life at least until the ninth decade. After age 90 the data are both scarce and considerably confounded. For example, persons with a tendency toward the development of Alzheimer's disease have a decreased life expectancy. Hence many of the people at greatest risk for the disease may be more likely to die before reaching the ninth or tenth decade. Weighing the available evidence, it is probably accurate to state that age is a major epidemiologic predisposing factor toward the development of Alzheimer's disease. As we shall see, even in the closest model for Alzheimer's disease, namely the dementia sometimes seen in persons with Down's syndrome, increasing age is strongly related to the development of the syndrome.

Can aging cause chromosomal breakage or damage?

Apparently it can. Many studies, beginning with that of Jacobs and his co-workers in 1961,[24] have found increased major chromosomal changes in aged tissues as compared with younger tissues. The most common tissue utilized in such investigations is white blood cells because of the relative ease with which they may be obtained. In dividing tissue such as white blood cells, chromosomal changes would be expected to accumulate over time and be passed on to future generations of cells. Neurons, of course, are different in that they do not divide over the course of the adult life span. Hence any changes in their genetic composition become permanent so long as the neurons remain alive. These special factors would appear to make neurons particularly vulnerable to traumatic genetic influences. A dividing tissue such as the white blood cells may simply "discard" a line of cells containing major genetic anomalies. The anomalous genetic line will die off and be replaced by cells from a relatively healthy ancestor. Obviously, a nondividing tissue such as the neuronal tissue does not have this option. However, a genuine compensation is the fact that cells are most vulnerable to traumatic genetic influences during the process of cellular division. Hence a nondividing cell such as a neuron is relatively impervious to many of the traumatic environmental influences—such as radiation—which would be most likely to cause chromosomal damage.

The current evidence is that neurons of elderly persons are more likely to show overt chromosomal changes than those of younger individuals. Furthermore, it is those same aged brains which have many neurons with broken or missing chromosomes which show the behavioral deficits of senile dementia.[18] Hence, there appears to be an interrelationship between aging, chromosomal damage, and Alzheimer's senile dementia.

The next element which we are postulating as a primary cause of Alzheimer's disease is "transmissible agents," or "viroids." We have already seen how the so-called "slow viruses" can produce dementias which are very similar clinically and pathologically to Alzheimer's disease. We have also referred to the emerging human evidence for a transmissible factor in at least some patients with Alzheimer's disease which was apparently capable of transmitting a very similar dementia condition to monkeys.

This evidence for a transmissible factor as a primary cause of Alzheimer's disease has recently been strengthened by investigations employing cultures of human nerve tissue. A factor extracted from the brains of Alzheimer's patients was capable of producing neurofilaments with the paired helical configuration characteristic of Alzheimer's disease in cell cultures of neurons from aborted human fetuses.[20] The factor, contained in a homogenate of Alzheimer's brain tissue, was active in inducing tangle formation even after being diluted up to 100,000 times. The factor was destroyed by heating. The factor was resistant to a DNA-destroying enzyme, but it was sensitive to RNA- and protein-destroying enzymes.

Hence the factor may be a virus. If it is a DNA virus, then it must be covered by a protective capsule which shields it from the DNA-destroying enzymes. Alternatively, the factor may be a virus containing RNA and protein. Classically, DNA viruses affect animals and RNA viruses attack plants. However, as we have seen, the slow viruses, which may be the closest relatives of the "Alzheimer's factor," are very unusual agents which have not yet been structurally identified. For example, the scrapie agent causes a slowly progressive degeneration of the central nervous system of sheep. The agent appears to have many unusual properties and continues to defy isolation. Among those unusual properties, the scrapie agent is apparently smaller than the smallest known animal (DNA) virus.[25] Hence it may be an RNA virus similar to the kind known to attack plants, or some new kind of transmissible virulent agent. RNA viruses have been implicated in the production of certain tumors in animals. Furthermore, similar viruses are known to cause chronic neurological diseases in both mice and sheep. Viruses which produce lymphatic tumors in mice also cause a paralytic disorder in those animals. Another RNA-like virus appears to cause chronic inflammation of the brains of sheep. For all these reasons, we are probably safer calling the slow viruses and the Alzheimer's transmissible factor "viroids" (virus-like agents) until more becomes known regarding their true nature.

Can viroids or viruses cause chromosomal changes?

Yes, in many ways. Viruses can locate themselves within the chromosomes themselves, employing the cellular genetic machinery for their own ends before ultimately breaking off and leaving a damaged chromosome in their wake. Viruses may also interfere with cellular chromosome maintenance and repair by their subversion of the cellular machinery.

Viroid and aging primary factors may combine to produce Alzheimer's disease. For example, chromosomal breakage and the resultant compromising of cellular resistance may trigger the activity of dormant viruses. It is likely that in all cases of Alzheimer's disease the two factors do indeed contribute jointly to the evolution of the pathology.

The third primary cause of Alzheimer's disease is heredito-familial factors. There is some evidence that Alzheimer's disease is more common among relatives of persons suffering from the condition. In the early 1960s systematic Scandinavian studies of hospital probands with senile dementia and their relatives within the community suggested that senile dementia is a disease that has a genetic basis.[26] Other investigations have uncovered families in which dementia of a relatively early onset is more likely to occur than is usual.[27] In this country, Leonard Heston and his associates at the University of Minnesota have conducted investigations which appear to have implicated familial factors in many cases of Alzheimer's disease.[28]

"Familial factors" does not necessarily imply a genetic basis per se. For example, hazards present in the environment which might result in chromosomal damage would be likely to be expressed in an increased incidence among persons coming from the same family. Similarly, infectious agents are more likely to spread to related persons whom an infected individual would be likely to have contact with than to unrelated strangers. It has been suggested that some of the slow virus conditions may have exceedingly long incubation periods, perhaps as long as several decades. If this were the case, these transmissible agents might cause an increased familial incidence even among siblings who had been separated for decades.

But regardless of the origins of the observed familial factors, a family history of Alzheimer's disease does appear to increase an individual's susceptibility to the disorder.

Down's syndrome, or mongolism, is a condition in which an extra chromosome is present in a specific part of the genome. Technically, it is also known as "trisomy G-21" because the third chromosome (trisomy) is presented on the 21st chromosomal "pair." The disease is remarkable as a model of senile dementia. One hundred percent of persons with Down's syndrome who survive into middle life develop a clinical and pathological condition identical to Alzheimer's disease![28,29]

Of course Down's sufferers generally have some impairment in their intellectual capacities, which is probably present at birth and which becomes manifest as retarded intellectual development during childhood. Completely apart from this general retardation or subnormality, Down's patients who survive into middle life begin to display signs of a dementia, most often in their thirties. They forget names of persons and things they have always known. They show the same kinds of early deficits as do persons in the early stages of senile dementia. Just as in Alzheimer's disease, these early cognitive deficits progress to a severe dementia with overt neurological and psychiatric symptoms as well as a severe intellectual deficit. Down's patients over 35 demonstrate a higher incidence of recent memory loss, short-term visual retention deficit, difficulty in object identification, loss of vocabulary, loss of affectionate responses toward others, and irritability and slowness with apparent loss of interest in their surroundings.[29] Neuropathological changes in the form of neurofibrillary tangles and senile plaques identical to those seen in Alzheimer's disease have been observed in *all* Down's patients over the age of 35 who come to autopsy.[30,31,32,33]

Other equally surprising interrelationships between Down's syndrome and Alzheimer's disease have been discovered. The incidence of Down's syndrome has been found to be increased in the families of persons with Alzheimer's presenile and senile dementia. In one study there were 6 persons with Down's syndrome among 777 persons born into Alzheimer's families.[28] Ordinarily, Down's syndrome occurs in about 1 in 700 live births. The probability of 6 Down's cases occurring by chance in the 777 births has been estimated as being less than 1 in 10,000. Furthermore, it is known that there is a 20-fold increase in the incidence of leukemia among persons with Down's syndrome. This increased incidence of leukemia apparently extends to the relatives of Down's patients. In a study of more than 3,000 parents of Down's syndrome patients, more than twice the expected rate of leukemia was found.[34] In the families of Alzheimer's disease patients, an increased incidence of blood cancer has also been found to occur.[28]

All of these conditions merge very neatly into our model of the origins of Alzheimer's disease. Apart from the characteristic chromosomal deficit in Down's syndrome in which the presence of an additional G-21 chromosome is diagnostic of the disorder, increased concentrations of chromosomal aberrations of different types have been reported in relatives of probands with trisomy D.[35] This is a congenital chromosomal abnormality less frequently encountered than Down's syndrome. Infants with trisomy D have an additional chromosome present in the so-called D group. The clinical picture is one of severe malformations centering in the facial structures and central nervous system. Similarly, leukemia has been reported to be associated with increased chromosomal aberrations.[36] Furthermore, apart from the evidence already discussed of the positive relationship between chromosomal abnormalities and clinical signs of overt dementia, there is indirect evidence for an increased incidence of chromosomal abnormalities in the *families* of Alzheimer's patients. In one study there appeared to be an increased incidence of congenital defects which suggests chromosomal aberrations among the families of Alzheimer's patients; also, neonatal deaths appeared to occur at approximately twice the expected rate in the families of Alzheimer's patients, another possible indicator of chromosomal abnormalities.[28]

Although these similarities and interrelationships between Down's syndrome, Alzheimer's disease, and leukemia are impressive, they do not account for the fact that all Down's sufferers ultimately develop a condition virtually identical to Alzheimer's disease. Evidently the genetic abnormality which is always present in Down's patients must, in and of itself, be sufficient cause for Alzheimer's disease. There are innumerable ways in which the presence of the extra chromosome might eventuate in the Alzheimer's syndrome. It might interfere directly with immunologic competence and neurotubular coding. Alternatively, it might produce substances which interfere with other chromosomes in such a way as to achieve the same results. Further speculations are possible but would be premature at this stage of our knowledge. However, it is clear that an increased understanding of Down's syndrome might ultimately lead to a solution of some of the remaining mysteries of Alzheimer's disease. It is one of nature's ironies that this congenital condition may help solve one of the great mysteries of the senium.

Next on our list of primary causes of Alzheimer's type senile dementia are toxic substances, such as metals. Among the latter, aluminum has been the most intensively studied in Alzheimer's disease. Several converging lines of evidence appear to indicate a primary etiologic role for aluminium in conjunction with other factors already described in the genesis of senile dementia.

Aluminum salt, injected into the brain of certain animals, including cats and rabbits, has induced a progressive dementia with neurofibrillary degeneration.[37] These animals displayed an initial loss of short-term memory and learning ability which was followed by loss of other brain functions.

In humans, the accumulation of aluminum and other metals in the central nervous system has long been known to be associated with dementia and encephalopathy. More recently, specific associations have been found. Aluminum has been strongly implicated in the dementia which occurs in patients receiving serum hemodialysis over an extended time course. In patients with kidney failure who were neither demented nor treated with dialysis, brain aluminum has been found more than seven times normal; in comparison, patients with dialysis dementia had mean brain aluminum concentrations which were more than fifteen times normal.[38]

Autopsies of the brains of persons with Alzheimer's disease have revealed an increased concentration of aluminum. Specifically, in six normal adults from 45 to 65 years of age, aluminum concentrations were 1.8 ± 0.7 $\mu g/g$ of tissue. In 16 brains of persons with Alzheimer's disease, concentrations up to 107 $\mu g/g$ of tissue were obtained. Of the brain regions surveyed in the Alzheimer's patients, 28 percent had concentrations greater than 4.0 $\mu g/g$. In two cases of dementia thought to be of vascular causation, brain tissue aluminum concentrations were comparable to those found in nondemented persons.[39]

The locations of the increased aluminum concentrations seen in the brains of Alzheimer's patients also are consistent with our theories of the origins of the disease. The increased aluminum concentrations appear to correspond with the areas of neurofibrillary degeneration. Concentrations are particularly high in and around the hippocampus. Within the neuron itself, the aluminum appears to concentrate within the nucleus and, even more specifically, within the chromosomal DNA material. In Alzheimer's disease, a three- to fourfold increase in aluminum content within the chromosomal material, as compared with controls, has been demonstrated.[40] Furthermore, there is some evidence that the neurotoxicity of aluminum may be the result of the interaction of this element with nuclear chromatin.[41] This, of course, would explain how aluminum, as a primary contributory factor to the development of Alzheimer's disease, produces the intermediate phase in which chromosomal breakage and altered transcription in general occurs.

However, the current evidence is that aluminum alone, without other contributory factors, does not produce true Alzheimer's disease. Neurofibrillary tangles which were induced in the brains of cats and rabbits by aluminum injections consisted of single-stranded filaments with a diameter of 100 Å.[39] The filaments lacked the helical configuration which we have described as one of the characteristic features of Alzheimer's disease. Furthermore, the induction process in human tissues appears to be very similar to that observed in other animals. Aluminum induced single-stranded, 100-Å neurofilaments in cell cultures of human neuronal tissue which were indistinguishable in appearance from those seen in cats or rabbits.[42] Even more convincing evidence that aluminum in the absence of other contributory factors does not produce Alzheimer's disease exists with respect to the other pathological features. Aluminum does not induce perivascular amyloid, nor the amyloid core of senile plaques. Neither does it produce the granulovacuolar degeneration seen in the hippocampal cells.

Other toxins in addition to aluminum have been shown to be capable of producing forms of neurofibrillary tangles. Some of those toxins may also contribute in some way to the development of Alzheimer's disease. An example of another metallic substance which has caused neurofibrillary degeneration is cadmium. Agents which interfere with cellular functioning by blocking cell division or protein synthesis have also caused tangle formation. However, thus far, only aluminum has been shown to induce a slowly progressive cerebral deterioration in conjunction with the development of the neurofibrillary tangles.

Hence we have seen how evidence from many different sources does produce a reasonably consistent model which can form a basis for our understanding of the origins and development of Alzheimer's disease, the major cause of senile dementia. For physicians and medical scientists this understanding must be translated into useful treatment approaches. Subsequently, we shall discuss work and progress in this crucial area. However, now that we have gone into great detail in the description of Alzheimer's disease, what about the other major, albeit less frequent causes of senile dementia?

Notes

1. Bowen, D. M., White, P., Spillane, J. A., Goodhardt, M. J., Curzon, G., Iwangoff, P., Meier-Ruge, W., and Davison, A. N., Accelerated ageing or selective neuronal loss as an important cause of dementia? *Lancet* i: 11–14, 1979.
2. Berger, B., Escourolle, R., and Moyne, M. A., Axones catécholaminergiques du cortex cérébral humain: Observation, en biofluorescence, de biopsies cérébrales dans 2 cas de maladie d'Alzheimer, *Rev. Neurol.* (Paris), 132: 183–194, 1976.
3. Winblad, B., Adolfsson, R., Gottfries, C. G., Oreland, L., and Roos, B. E., Brain monoamines, monoamine metabolites and enzymes in physiological ageing and senile dementia. In *Recent Advances in Mass Spectrometry in Biochemistry and Medicine,* ed. by A. Frigerio, 1978, vol. 1 pp. 253–267.

4. Innes, I. R., and Nickerson, N., Drugs inhibiting the action of acetylcholine on structures innervated by postganglionic parasympathetic nerves (antimuscarinic or atropinic drugs). In Gilman, A. G., Goodman, L. S., and Gilman, A. (eds.), *The Pharmacological Basis of Therapeutics;* 4th ed., Macmillan, New York, 1970, pp. 524-548.

5. Drachman, D. A., and Leavitt, J., Human memory and the cholinergic system: A relationship to aging. *Arch. Neurol.* 30: 113-121, 1974.

6. Davis, K. L., Hollister, L. E., Overall, J., Johnson, A., and Train, K., Physostigmine: Effects on cognition and affect in normal subjects. *Psychopharmacology* 51:23-27, 1976.

7. Schmidt, L. F., *The Cerebral Circulation in Health and Disease,* Thomas, Springfield, Ill., 1950.

8. Ingvar, D. H., and Gustafson, L., Regional cerebral blood flow in organic dementia with early onset. *Acta Neurol. Scand.* 43: 42-73, 1970.

9. Obrist, W. D., Chivian, E., Cronquist, S., and Ingvar, D. H., Regional cerebral blood flow in senile and presenile dementia. *Neurology* (Minneapolis) 20: 315-322, 1970.

10. Ingvar, D. H., Brun, A., Hagberg, B., and Gustafson, L., Regional cerebral blood flow in the dominant hemisphere in confirmed cases of Alzheimer's disease, Pick's disease, and multi-infarct dementia: Relationship to clinical symptomatology and neuropathological findings. In R. Katzman, R. D. Terry, and K. L. Bick (eds.), *Alzheimer's Disease: Senile Dementia and Related Disorders (Aging,* Vol. 7), Raven Press, New York, 1978.

11. Obrist, W. D., Thompson, H. K., Jr., Wang, H. S., and Wilkinson, W. E., Regional cerebral blood flow estimated by xenon[133] inhalation. *Stroke* 6: 245-256, 1975.

12. Gustafson, L., Hagberg, B., and Ingvar, D. H., Speech disturbances in presenile dementia related to local cerebral blood flow abnormalities in the dominant hemisphere. *Brain Language* 5: 103-118, 1978.

13. Blass, J. P., Metabolic dementias. International Society for Neurochemistry Satellite Meeting on Aging of the Brain and Dementia, Florence, Aug. 27-29, 1979, Abstract, p. 66.

14. Bartus, R., Dean, R., and Goas, J., Anoxia-induced amnesia as a neuropsychopharmacologic model of aging. Presented at American Aging Association, 9th Annual Meeting, Washington, D.C., Sept. 20-22, 1979.

15. Nielson, J., Chromosomes in senile dementia. *Brit. J. Psychiat.* 115: 303-309, 1968.

16. Jarvik, L. F., and Kato, T., Chromosomes and mental changes in octogenarians: Preliminary findings. *Brit. J. Psychiat.* 115: 1193-1194, 1969.

17. Jarvik, L. F., Altshuler, K. Z., Kato, T., and Blumner, B., Organic

brain syndrome and chromosome loss in aged twins. *Diseases of the Nervous System* 32: 159–170, 1971.

18. Jarvik, L. F., Memory loss and its possible relationship to chromosome changes. In *Advances in Behavioral Biology,* Vol. 6, ed. by C. Eisdorfer and W. E. Fann, Plenum Press, New York–London, 1973, pp. 145–150.

19. Fischman, H. K., Albu, P., Reisberg, B., Ferris, S., and Rainer, J. D., Elevation of sister chromatid exchanges in female Alzheimer's disease. Presented at the American Society of Human Genetics, New York, September 1980.

20. Crapper, D. R., and De Boni, U., Etiological factors in dementia. Presented at the International Society for Neurochemistry Satellite Meeting on Aging of the Brain and Dementia, Florence, Aug. 27–29, 1979.

21. Iqbal, K., Neurofibrous proteins in aging and dementia. Presented at the International Society for Neurochemistry Satellite Meeting on Aging of the Brain and Dementia, Florence, Aug. 27–29, 1979.

22. Nandy, K., Immune reactions in aging brain and senile dementia. In *The Aging Brain and Senile Dementia,* Vol. 23 in *Advances in Behavioral Biology,* ed. by K. Nandy and I. Sherwin, 1977, pp. 181–196.

23. Nandy, K., Brain-reactive antibodies in aging and senile dementia. In *Alzheimer's Disease: Senile Dementia and Related Disorders (Aging,* Vol. 7), ed. by R. Katzman, R. D. Terry, and K. L. Bick, Raven Press, New York, 1978.

24. Jacobs, P. A., Court Brown, W. M., and Doll, R., Distribution of human chromosome counts in relation to age. *Nature* (London) 197: 1178–1180, 1961.

25. Prusiner, S. B., Hadlow, W. J., Groth, D. C., Race, R. E., and Cochran, S. P., Free flow electrophoresis and gradient centrifugation of the scrapie agent. International Society for Neurochemistry Satellite Meeting on Aging of the Brain and Dementia, Florence, Aug. 27–29, 1979, Abstracts, p. 50.

26. Larsson, T., Sjogren, T., and Jacobsen, G., Senile dementia. *Acta Psychiat. Scand.* 39: Suppl. 167, 1963.

27. Wheelan, Lorna, Familial Alzheimer's disease. *Ann. Hum. Genet.* 23: 300–310, 1957.

28. Heston, L. L., and Mastri, A. R., The genetics of Alzheimer's disease. *Arch. Gen. Psychiat.* 34: 976–981, 1977.

29. Wisniewski, K., Howe, J., Williams, G. D., and Wisniewski, H. M., Precocious aging and dementia in patients with Down's syndrome. *Biol. Psychiat.,* Vol. 18, No. 5, 619–627, 1978.

30. Struwe, F., Histopathological Untersuch ugen uber Einstehrungen und Wesen stech der senile Plaques. *Z. Ges. Neurol. Psychiat.* 122: 291, 1929.

31. Jervis, G. A., Early senile dementia in mongoloid idiocy. *Amer. J. Psychiat.* 105: 102, 1948.

32. Olson, M. I., and Shaw, C. M., Presenile dementia and Alzheimer's disease in mongolism. *Brain* 92: 147–156, 1969.

33. Crapper, D. R., Dalton, A. L., Skopitz, M., Eng, P., Scott, J. H., and Hachinski, V., Alzheimer's degeneration in Down's syndrome. *Arch. Neurol.* 32: 618, 1975.

34. Holland, W. W., Doll, R., and Carter, C. O., The mortality from leukemia and other cancers among patients with Down's syndrome (mongols) and among their parents. *Brit. J. Cancer* 16: 177–186, 1962.

35. Hecht, F., Bryant, J. S., Gruber, D., et al., The nonrandomness of chromosomal abnormalities. Association of trisomy 18 and Down's syndrome. *New England J. Med.* 271: 1081–1086, 1964.

36. Miller, R. W., Down's syndrome (mongolism), other congenital malformations and cancers among the sibs of leukemic children. *New England J. Med.* 268: 393–401, 1963.

37. Klatzo, I., Wisniewski, H., and Streicher, E., Experimental production of neurofibrillary degeneration. *J. Neuropath. Exp. Neurol.* 24: 187–199, 1965.

38. Arieff, A. I., Cooper, J. D., Armstrong, D., and Lazarowitz, V. C., Dementia, renal failure, and brain aluminum. *Ann. Intern. Med.* 90: 741, 1979.

39. Crapper, D. R., Functional consequences of neurofibrillary degeneration. In *Neurobiology of Aging,* ed. by R. D. Terry and S. Gershon, Raven Press, New York, 1976, pp. 405–432.

40. Crapper, D. R., Karlik, S., and De Boni, U., Aluminum and other metals in senile (Alzheimer) dementia. In *Alzheimer's Disease: Senile Dementia and Related Disorders (Aging,* Vol. 7), ed. by R. Katzman, R. D. Terry, and K. L. Bick, Raven Press, New York, 1978, pp. 471–485.

41. De Boni, U., Seger, M., and Crapper, D., Interaction of aluminum and chromatin in human cells in vitro as assessed by DNA-repair. Presented at American Aging Association, 9th Annual Meeting, Washington, D.C., Sept. 20–22, 1979.

42. De Boni, U., Dalton, A. J., Schlotterer, G., and Crapper, D. R., Senile dementia: Recent concepts of pathophysiology. In *Research in Dementia: Proceedings of a Colloquium of the Ontario Psycho-Geriatric Association,* Research Bulletin, Vol. 3, No. 1, 1–15, June 1977.

Chapter 4

Late Life Dementia: The Other Causes of Senility

ALZHEIMER'S DISEASE APPEARS TO BE the source of the majority of late life dementias. But what of the remainder? What are the other origins of senile brain failure?

The classical autopsy studies of the English investigators Tomlinson, Blessed, and Roth once again provide the initial findings from which much of our understanding of the causes of dementia originates. It will be recalled that this team followed 50 demented persons from the period of their illness to their demise. They then investigated the brains of these persons, comparing them with controls of similar age.[1,2] As we have said, in the majority of cases the pathology indicated an Alzheimer's disease process. In 9 of the 50 cases, however, there were no significant findings of plaques or tangles. Instead these 9 dementia cases had multiple areas of what the pathologists called "cerebral softening." By this they meant degenerated and hemorrhagic brain tissue which they recognized as a result of the blockage of cerebral blood vessels. In demented persons without any evidence of Alzheimer's disease, the volume of brain tissue with the so-called "cerebral softening" was positively related to the presence of dementia.

Tomlinson, Blessed, and Roth also distinguished a third group of demented patients, comprising approximately a quarter of the total

63

sample, in whom "mixed" pathology was discovered upon autopsy. This "mixed" group had a combination of Alzheimer's pathology *and* areas of cerebral softening.

Thus this second major source of senility, characterized by what pathologists descriptively call cerebral softening, appears to be the major cause of approximately 15 percent of all late life dementias, and appears to contribute, together with Alzheimer's disease, to another 25 percent of senile dementias. Because of our belief that the cerebral softening is the product of multiple cerebral infarctions which accumulate over time, the term "multi-infarct dementia" (M.I.D.) has been suggested for this second major entity.[3]

Current evidence indicates that the source of the cerebral infarctions which accumulate to produce M.I.D. is generally material from atherosclerotic vessels *outside* the brain. Hence, in reference to patients with this second major cause of senility, M.I.D., and in reference to patients with "mixed" dementia in which M.I.D. is a contributory factor, there was an element of truth to the former conceptions of arteriosclerotic causation. However, our current understanding of M.I.D. is quite different in detail from the former theories. The pathological findings of Corsellis and his successors, referred to in earlier chapters, have taught us that *cerebral* arteriosclerosis is not the cause of any commonly occurring dementia, including M.I.D.; however, *peripheral* arteriosclerosis in the heart, the extremities, and the remainder of the cardiovascular system does predispose to M.I.D. Nor is it progressively narrowed arteriosclerotic cerebral vessels which result in dementia; rather, it is the progressive accumulation of cerebral infarctions, large and small, and the resultant diffuse destruction of brain tissue.

All of the conditions which predispose toward cardiovascular arteriosclerosis are associated with an increased incidence and severity of M.I.D. These risk factors include (1) myocardial infarction (heart attacks), angina pectoris (severe chest pains), and other cardiac conditions in which arteriosclerosis is a contributing factor, (2) hypertension (high blood pressure), (3) so-called "transient ischemic attacks" (TIAs),* (4) peripheral vascular disease with "coldness," "tingling,"

---

* These are short-lasting episodes of focal cerebral dysfunction generally resulting from a cerebral embolus or infarction. The most frequent symptoms are temporary sensory disturbances or weakening of the arms or legs, together with speech problems or loss of vision in one eye. These symptoms are sometimes accompanied by fainting, confusion, dizziness, or a spinning sensation. Often these episodes last only 5 to 10 minutes, and three-quarters of TIAs are over within an hour.[4]

"numbness," "pain," and other abnormal sensations in the arms and legs (and especially the fingers and toes), (5) diabetes mellitus ("sugar diabetes"), (6) obesity, and, to a lesser extent, (7) cigarette smoking. These factors point to obvious treatment implications for this form of dementia, which will be discussed in a later chapter.

What is the course of M.I.D.? Can it be distinguished from Alzheimer's disease, or do these very different causes result in precisely the same condition?

Apparently the two forms of dementia are quite dissimilar. Alzheimer's disease is a slow, progressive condition. M.I.D. appears to be abrupt in onset and episodic in course, with numerous remissions and exacerbations. We can diagram these differences as in Figure 4–1, recognizing that the slopes refer to averaged, typical cases and would not adequately describe many demented and confused individuals.

The conditions differ in presentation as well as in course. Because Alzheimer's disease tends to affect roughly the same areas of the brain and tends to be symmetrical, that is, to occur to approximately the same extent on both sides of the brain, it has a fairly uniform course and presentation. These will be discussed in detail in subsequent chapters. M.I.D. is much more variable in its clinical appearance, as well as its course. This is quite logical if we consider that M.I.D. is the result of emboli, large and small, which occur at various times and

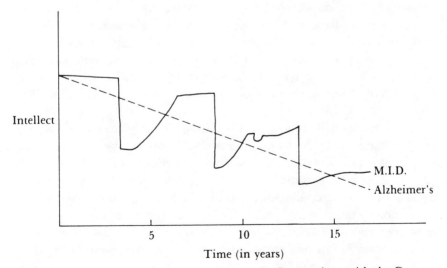

Figure 4.1 Course of Alzheimer's Disease in Comparison with the Course of Multi-infarct Dementia

which may affect very different brain areas. Hence M.I.D. frequently results in what neurologists refer to as "focal signs," that is, pathology which can be recognized as originating from a particular area of the brain. It is believed that true dementia does not occur unless the destruction affects both halves of the brain. It is probably also true that infarctions in M.I.D. would have to affect the hippocampi on both sides of the brain for the characteristic Alzheimer's-like deficit in recent memory to occur.

There are many other ways in which M.I.D. differs from Alzheimer's dementia. For instance, the incidence of Alzheimer's disease appears to increase steadily from early middle age to old age, and perhaps throughout life. In contrast, the incidence of M.I.D. is said to parallel that of stroke and may peak at from 40 to 60 years of age. There are numerous epidemiologic distinctions. In the case of M.I.D., the incidence is strongly associated with the presence of cardiovascular arteriosclerosis. The "risk factors" for cardiovascular arteriosclerosis are also risk factors for M.I.D. One risk factor which has not yet been mentioned is sex. Men are more likely to be affected by M.I.D. For Alzheimer's the relative sex incidence appears to be equal.[5]

Pathologically, of course, the conditions are quite dissimilar. M.I.D. appears as asymmetric, diffuse, irregular areas of cerebral softening. Occasionally there is evidence of cerebral infarction and embolization. Outside the brain there is virtually always evidence of arteriosclerotic disease. As we have said, in Alzheimer's disease the pathology consists of the characteristic neurofibrillary tangles, senile plaques, and granulovacuolar degeneration, appearing symmetrically in the cortex. The more subtle Alzheimer's pathological changes such as preferential loss of cholinergic neurons in certain brain regions are also absent in M.I.D.

Immunologically, biochemically, and genetically the conditions are also distinguishable. M.I.D. patients would not be expected to display the increase in brain-reactive antibodies, the decrease in CAT activity, or the increased chromosomal breakage described in Alzheimer's disease. Specialized diagnostic tools such as computerized axial tomographic brain scans and radioisotope studies of cerebral blood flow may also reveal differences in the two conditions (see Table 4–1 for a summary of the distinctions between these two common forms of dementia in the aged).

We have said that more than half of the dementias of late life ap-

TABLE 4-1.   Distinctions between Multi-Infarct Dementia (M.I.D.) and Alzheimer's Disease, the two most frequent causes of dementia and intellectual decline in the elderly

	M.I.D.	ALZHEIMER'S DISEASE
1. Onset	May be abrupt	Insidious
2. Course	Stepwise and paroxysmal	Gradual and progressive
3. Sex	Men more frequent	Equally distributed
4. Neurological focal signs	Frequent	Generally absent
5. Pathology at autopsy	Cerebral softening with multiple areas of infarction; cardiovascular arteriosclerosis	Neurofibrillary tangles, senile plaques; granulovacuolar degeneration; increased dendritic spine loss
6. Associated medical pathology	Strokes and other cerebral vascular accidents; myocardial infarctions, angina pectoris, and other cardiac pathology; hypertension; TIAs; peripheral vascular disease, diabetes mellitus; obesity	Increased familial incidence of Down's syndrome and leukemia
7. Autoimmunity	Normal brain-reactive antibodies	Increased brain-reactive antibodies for age
8. Genetic	No increased incidence of chromosomal breakage	Increased incidence of chromosomal breakage proportional to severity of the dementia
9. Biochemical	No change in brain CAT activity	CAT activity inversely proportional to severity of memory impairment
10. Diagnostic tools		
a. CT scans	Focal and asymmetric pathology	Symmetrical atrophy and ventricular enlargement related to severity of the dementia
b. Xenon 133 radioisotope studies of cerebral blood flow, with CO_2 enhancement	None or decreased blood flow	Increased blood flow compared with age-matched controls
11. Treatment	Aspirin and agents which decrease platelet aggregation and clotting; Antihypertensives; Possibly anticoagulants	Cerebral vasodilators and metabolic enhancers; neurotransmitters; neuropeptides, etc.

pear to be the result of Alzheimer's disease alone, approximately 15 percent appear to be the result of M.I.D., and perhaps 25 percent are from a combination of M.I.D. and Alzheimer's disease. This leaves us with approximately 10 percent of the late life dementias of formerly unknown causation unaccounted for. We now know that a large fraction of these remaining dementias are the result of psychiatric depression, an entity sometimes referred to as "pseudodementia."*,6

A full discussion of depression is beyond the scope of the book. However, depression is a common illness in the elderly. In one study of persons attending an information and counseling service for older persons, almost 40 percent of the elderly people had a form of depressive illness.[7] In another study of persons in a mental health program for elderly outpatients, more than half of the patients had depressive illness.[8] Surveys of the elderly in private psychiatric inpatient facilities similarly reveal one-third to one-half of the patients to have depression.[9,10]

Depression is marked by symptoms including low self-esteem, anxiety, agitation, social withdrawal, feelings of guilt, difficulty sleeping, loss of appetite, weight loss, crying spells, loss of energy, fatigue, pessimism, headaches, dizziness, and hypochondriacal symptoms. Many of these symptoms, alone and in combination, are associated with a decrease in memory and intellect. For example, in a subsequent chapter we will discuss the similarity between the impairment of memory and intellect produced by anxiety and that observed in the early stage of Alzheimer's disease. Additionally, depressed people tend to exaggerate their deficits and to emphasize weaknesses in their capacities in general, even where such weaknesses may not be real. Depressed persons have a slowing of movement and of speech. Accompanying these is a slowing of thought. Anxiety, low self-esteem, underestimation of one's true capacities, and generalized slowing result in the "pseudodementia" of depression.

Some investigators have found a deficit in short-term memory in depressed persons without impairment of long-term memory.[11] However, other authors emphasize the variability and inconsistency of

---

* "Pseudodementia," strictly speaking, refers to an "organic brain syndrome" or intellectual disturbance which is the result of a primary "functional" disturbance. "Functional" disturbances would include psychoses and certain other kinds of psychiatric disturbances as well as depression. However, depression is said to be the most frequent cause of pseudodementia,[6] and the two terms are sometimes used interchangeably.

the depressed person's cognitive impairment,[12] and this latter description is more consistent with clinical experience.

Depressed patients frequently exaggerate the extent of their intellectual deficit. In distinction, Alzheimer's patients show realistic concern in regard to their decrease in memory capacity during the very early stage of their condition. Once their deficit becomes recognizable to others, Alzheimer's patients tend to deny their condition. The denial in Alzheimer's patients can be readily distinguished from the depressed patient's exaggeration. Hence memory and intellectual impairment associated with primary depressive illness can generally be recognized by the experienced clinician. The presence of other elements in the depressive syndrome, the exaggeration of deficit, and inconsistencies in the deficit are clues to the diagnosis. When memory and intellectual impairment is the result of depressive illness, treatment of the latter results in improvement in cognition.[11]

Depression may also exist together with Alzheimer's disease in elderly persons. Anxiety and depression are particularly common in the latter stages of Alzheimer's disease when the degree of deficit becomes so large that psychological defense mechanisms no longer enable patients to entirely deny their condition. Chemical and neurotransmitter changes in the late stages of Alzheimer's disease may also predispose toward depression.

When depression exists in association with Alzheimer's disease, the depression is responsive to standard antidepressant treatments. However, the memory and intellectual deficits which are secondary to Alzheimer's disease remain after the depression has resolved.[13]

Another cause of dementia in the elderly which has only recently been seen to be of considerable magnitude and influence is Parkinson's disease. Because the primary Parkinsonian condition is the one most frequently diagnosed, both during life and at autopsy, the incidence of this dementia in the elderly is not reflected in the statistics which have been discussed earlier.

Parkinsonism has already been mentioned more than once in our account of the origins of Alzheimer's disease. We have discussed the presence of neurofibrillary tangles identical to those found in Alzheimer's disease in the brains of persons with certain kinds of Parkinsonian syndromes. Specifically, we have noted that PHFs are present in the postencephalitic Parkinsonian syndrome of viral causation and in the hereditary Parkinsonian syndrome which occurs among the Chamorro people on the island of Guam. PHFs are also present in dementia pugilistica, a condition resulting from repeated head injuries in which a Parkinsonian syndrome is frequently observed.

In all of these Parkinsonian conditions, the PHFs have been said to be located primarily in the substantia nigra, the area of the brain which has been most closely identified with Parkinsonian pathology, rather than in the hippocampus, as are the PHFs of Alzheimer's disease.

As discussed earlier, Parkinsonism is a syndrome, or cluster of symptoms which tend to occur together and which represent a "final common pathway" which may be the result of a variety of causative conditions. The most frequent condition which results in the Parkinsonian syndrome is of unknown origin at this time. This common form of Parkinsonism is known as "primary" or "idiopathic" Parkinsonism.

Classically, dementia, or "general mental deterioration," was not recognized as an important component of primary Parkinsonism. Even after its presence came to be recognized, it was thought to occur infrequently, and the association between the two conditions has not been emphasized.[14,15] However, studies conducted over the past several years have found that from 20 to 80 percent of primary Parkinsonian patients have notable mental deterioration.[16,17,18,19,20,21] Since 375,000 Americans are estimated to have clinically significant primary Parkinsonism and it has been estimated that one in every forty persons will develop the condition during his or her lifetime,[15] the number of persons with dementia associated with this condition is certainly not inconsiderable.

In a study of over 500 patients with Parkinsonism conducted at the New York University Medical Center, approximately one-third were found to have moderate to marked dementia. This was 10 times the incidence of dementia in the spouses of the Parkinsonian patients. Furthermore, the Parkinsonian patients with dementia were found to differ from the Parkinsonian patients without dementia in certain important characteristics. Parkinsonian patients with dementia were older and developed the Parkinsonian syndrome later in life than did nondemented Parkinsonian patients. Also, the Parkinsonian syndrome appears to progress more rapidly in persons with accompanying intellectual impairment than in Parkinsonian patients of normal intellect. Finally, the classic Parkinsonian therapy, levodopa (L-dopa), appears to be less effective in Parkinsonian patients with accompanying dementia than in those without cognitive decline. On the basis of these findings, it has recently been suggested that primary Parkinsonism with dementia may represent a different disorder than primary Parkinsonism without dementia.[22]

We know that Parkinsonian syndromes of diverse origin are all characterized by common pathological findings which can be demonstrated in the brain at the time of autopsy. These common findings include loss of pigment and accompanying degenerative changes in the part of the brain known as the substantia nigra. We have seen that certain of the less frequent causes of the Parkinsonian syndrome are also accompanied by other kinds of brain pathology including neurofibrillary tangles of the Alzheimer's type. What kinds of brain pathology are observed when autopsies are conducted on persons who had suffered from primary Parkinsonism and dementia?

Until very recently, answers to this logical query were either unsatisfactory or unavailable. However, in conducting an autopsy on a patient with Parkinson's disease and progressive dementia, Hakim and Mathieson at the Montreal Neurological Institute found changes in the brain characteristic of both Parkinson's disease and Alzheimer's disease. This prompted them to do a retrospective review of the brain findings in Parkinsonian patients in comparison with controls. Their findings are somewhat astounding. Fifty-six percent of the 34 Parkinson's disease patients whom they studied retrospectively had shown some dementia symptomatology. Senile plaques were noted in the hippocampal portions of the brain in 29 of the 34 cases of Parkinson's disease. In comparison, senile plaques were observed in the hippocampus in only 5 of 34 age-matched control brains which came from patients who had died of cerebral infarction or trauma. Analogously, neurofibrillary tangles were found in the hippocampi in 29 of the Parkinson's cases and in only 7 of the controls. Granulovacuolar degeneration was observed in the hippocampal neurons in 30 of the Parkinsonian's brains in comparison with 7 of the control brains. Twenty-seven of the Parkinsonian cases were thought to have demonstrable cell loss in the neocortex. Neocortical cell loss was thought to have been present in 15 of the controls. Only one Parkinsonian case appeared to be free of all of the neuropathological changes which are usually associated with Alzheimer's disease.[23,24]

Hence the dementia found in association with Parkinson's disease, formerly unknown, is now recognized to be a major entity, probably causing moderate to severe impairment in more than 100,000 Americans. Furthermore, this dementia appears to be identical neuropathologically to Alzheimer's disease. Idiopathic Parkinsonism must predispose in some as yet unknown way toward the development of Alzheimer's neuropathological changes. Whether the dementia associated with Parkinson's disease is identical to senile dementia of the Alzheimer's type in other ways such as course and treatment is as yet unknown. However, we must now classify primary Parkinson's disease with Down's syndrome (mongolism) as an entity associated both with dementia and with neuropathological findings identical to those observed in S.D.A.T. As is the case in Down's syndrome and in S.D.A.T., the dementia in primary Parkinsonism appears to become more frequent with increasing age.

If Parkinson's disease is associated with Alzheimer's clinical and neuropathological findings, is the converse true? In other words, are Parkinsonian clinical and neuropathological findings observed more frequently in persons with Alzheimer's disease? Clinically, the tentative answer appears to be "somewhat more frequently." In aged patients with mild to moderate memory impairment, we found a slight increase in symptoms associated with Parkinsonism, with increasing magnitude of cognitive decline.[25] However, the majority of our patients did not display any of the "extrapyramidal symptoms" that we associate with Parkinsonism, and those patients who were symptomatic displayed only mild Parkinsonian symptomatology. Pathologically, in patients with severe Alzheimer's disease, some very interesting findings have been reported. The presence of large numbers of hyaline inclusion bodies in the cells of the substantia nigra and other primary sites of Parkinson's disease pathology is one of the most characteristic features of primary, or idiopathic, Parkinson's disease.[15,26] These hyaline inclusion bodies are most frequently referred to as "Lewy bodies." Large numbers of Lewy bodies have been so closely associated with idiopathic Parkinson's disease that some investigators have suggested that the presence of this pathology in "non-Parkinsonian" individuals probably represents a "preclinical" form of Parkinson's disease.[26,27] Lewy bodies have been found in 10 percent of 96 brains with Alzheimer's disease. In a control group of 77 persons of comparable age without dementia or Parkinsonian symptoms, Lewy bodies were not identified in any individual.[28] These preliminary findings certainly need to be expanded. They do, however, suggest that there might be an association between Alzheimer's brain pathology and certain kinds of pathology ordinarily associated with idiopathic Parkinson's disease just as an association has been found between

Parkinsonian brain pathology and the pathognomonic features of Alzheimer's disease.

Another cause of adult dementia is a recently described condition associated with progressive dementia known as normal pressure hydrocephalus (NPH). Normal pressure hydrocephalus was first identified by Hakim and Adams in 1965.[29] It is a clinical syndrome characterized by a gait disturbance and urinary incontinence in addition to a slowly progressive dementia. The diagnosis is confirmed by techniques which enable clinicians to visualize the brain's surfaces, including the fluid-filled cavities on the inner surface of the brain. These fluid-filled cavities contain the cerebral spinal fluid, or CSF, the liquid mixture which bathes the brain. The inner brain cavities are known as the cerebral ventricles. A succession of modern technologies, many of which involve the use of radioisotopes, have enabled clinicians to reconstruct pictures of these cavities within the brain and to estimate their size. In NPH the ventricles on the inside of the brain are found to be enlarged.

The fluid surrounding the brain is in a dynamic state; that is to say, the fluid is constantly changing. New fluid is continuously secreted by the brain, and the fluid which is already present is continuously drained off into the general circulation. Any condition which interferes with the drainage of the cerebral fluid, such as a tumor, bleeding, or injury to the brain substance, will ordinarily result in a build-up in pressure in the CSF. If the outflow of the CSF is blocked for a long period of time, this increase of pressure will cause the cerebral substance to become compressed and the cerebral ventricles to become enlarged. In normal pressure hydrocephalus the cerebral ventricles are enlarged; however, the pressure of the cerebral spinal fluid is normal. Most physicians who have worked with NPH patients have assumed that the reason the CSF pressure is normal in this condition is that compensatory compression of the brain, expansion of the cerebral ventricles, and, perhaps, decrease in production of CSF have collectively worked to restore the CSF pressure to normal over an extended period of time.

Frequently, the cause of NPH can be identified. In these cases the presence of a hemorrhagic condition, of a tumor, or of some other obstruction provides a ready explanation for the condition. In other cases, however, no obvious cause for the condition can be identified, and in these cases the condition has been termed idiopathic NPH. It is this idiopathic NPH which must be distinguished from Alzheimer's disease and other causes of dementia occurring in middle and late life.

The distinction between idiopathic NPH, with dilated cerebral ventricles and a progressive dementia, and Alzheimer's disease may be rendered particularly difficult, since enlarged cerebral ventricles are present in conjunction with a progressive dementia in the latter condition as well. In Alzheimer's disease, as we have seen, parts of the cortex, or outer layers, of the brain gradually decay. This process is accompanied by enlargement of the cerebral ventricles and deepening of the grooves, known as the sulci, on the outer layers of the brain. The most effective diagnostic tool currently available for visualizing changes in the brain substance in living persons is the computerized tomographic, or CT, scan, referred to earlier. Initial attempts to establish a relationship between ventricular enlargement and cortical atrophy as visualized on CT scans and clinical assessments of the severity of cognitive impairment in Alzheimer's disease were for the most part unsuccessful.[30,31,32] Lack of clarity in the initial generations of tomographic scanners, difficulties associated with comparing ventricular dilatation and cortical atrophy in different individuals with different head sizes and brain contours, and variability in the location of CT brain "slices" all contributed to the initial failures to find the expected associations. More recently, using comparative techniques, my associates and I at the New York University Medical Center have found a strong relationship between the extent of enlargement of the cerebral ventricles and the degree of cognitive impairment in persons with mild to moderately severe Alzheimer's disease.[33,34,35] Is idiopathic NPH, which like Alzheimer's is characterized by dilated cerebral ventricles, normal CSF pressure, and progressive dementia, and which unlike typical Alzheimer's disease has the additional clinical features of gait disturbance and urinary incontinence, then simply an atypical variant of Alzheimer's disease? Because biopsies as well as autopsies have occasionally been conducted on persons with idiopathic NPH, a fairly satisfactory answer to this question is available. For the answer to be meaningful, however, we must describe the syndrome of NPH in further detail.

The syndrome of idiopathic NPH first described by Adams and his co-workers[36] does not appear to be common. Although the condition has most frequently been noted to occur in the presenium, it appears to comprise only approximately one-twentieth of all cases of juvenile dementia, even when specifically sought.[37,38,39] The treatment for idiopathic NPH which has been consistently advocated since the initial description of the disorder is a neurosurgical procedure known as "shunting." This consists of the placement of an artificial device in the brain cavity to assist in the drainage of the cerebrospinal fluid. In idiopathic NPH approximately 40 percent of all patients operated upon have responded favorably to this procedure.[40] The brain surgery itself is not without risk, and from 6 to 9 percent of patients in whom the procedure has been tried have been reported to have died.[41,42] Shunt-related complications, occasionally requiring a repeat surgical procedure, have been reported in approximately 40 percent of patients operated upon. Hence, although idiopathic NPH is an uncommon condition, the proper diagnosis and treatment of the disorder are certainly of more than academic interest.

From what we have already said regarding adult dementia, there is one other set of dementias which might account for the variability in clinical course and response to therapy seen in idiopathic NPH. This other dementia type would also account for some of the specific clinical symptoms and the dilated cerebral ventricles with normal CSF pressure, observed in NPH. This other dementia set also appears to occur in the presenium more frequently than in older age groups—the other dementias to which I am referring are the vascular dementias such as M.I.D. Indeed, in three idiopathic NPH patients who had a positive response to surgical shunting, two had biopsies which revealed vascular changes consistent with hypertension. The authors who reported this reported 12 biopsies in patients who failed to respond to shunt therapy. Six of these therapy failures had Alzheimer's brain changes, three showed nonspecific cortical atrophy, and in three the biopsies were normal.[43]

Hence current information with respect to idiopathic NPH is that it is a clinical syndrome which may be the result of more frequently occurring and better-known causes of dementia including Alzheimer's disease and M.I.D. The variability in response to neurosurgical intervention, with frequent subsequent decline, may be accounted for by "a spontaneous remission coincidental with surgery, as often occurs in patients with vascular disease."[39]

The other causes of senile dementia discussed in this chapter—multi-infarct dementia, depression, idiopathic Parkinsonism, and idiopathic NPH—are all in their own ways inextricably bound to the story of Alzheimer's disease itself. Other causes of dementia alluded to earlier in our discussion also have touched upon our description of the origins of Alzheimer's disease. For example, certain viral conditions which produce an inflammation of the brain (encephalitis) and resultant dementia have been shown to relate pathologically, and perhaps in other ways as well, to Alzheimer's disease. The encephalitides which result from "slow virus" infections, notably kuru and Creutzfeldt-Jakob disease, appear to be particularly closely related, in terms of the kinds of changes which they produce in the brain, to Alzheimer's disease. Specific toxic causes of dementia, such as aluminium poisoning, have also been shown to produce certain kinds of brain changes which are analogous to certain changes found in Alzheimer's disease. There are numerous other possible causes of dementia which have not yet been linked to Alzheimer's disease apart from the obvious necessity for diagnosticians to distinguish between the diverse causes so that proper therapeutic measures can be instituted and an appropriate prognosis can be formulated.

Some of these other causes of dementia will probably be found to be more closely related to Alzheimer's disease in other significant ways in the near future. For example, Huntington's disease is a hereditary dementia of middle life which is characterized by abnormal "jerking movements," which generally appear before the onset of mental changes. Changes in the brain's neurotransmitter systems, including a decrease in CAT activity in affected portions of the brain, have been described in Huntington's disease.[44] Perhaps other kinds of pathological changes more closely associated with Alzheimer's disease will eventually be found in this disorder.

The possible causes of dementia, or generalized cerebral dysfunction, span the entire range of medical etiologies. Dementias can result from traumatic causes, from tumors, from vascular disease, from metabolic disorders, from external toxins, from hereditary conditions, from nutritional deficiencies, from infectious disorders, from endocrine disturbances, or from "unknown causes." A detailed description of the more common of the innumerable possible causes of dementia can be found in standard medical texts. Given this tremendous variety, how can a physician arrive at a diagnosis of Alzheimer's disease with reasonable certainty?

Pathologically, we can still make the statement that Alzheimer's disease is the *only* disease of adult life in which large numbers of PHFs and neuritic plaques are found in the neocortex in the absence of pathological changes in the basal ganglia and other deeper brain structures.

Clinically, Alzheimer's disease remains a "diagnosis of exclusion" during an individual's lifetime. A physician is obligated to consider a diagnosis of Alzheimer's disease in any patient with slowly progressive intellectual impairment occurring in middle or late life. However, the physician must also consider all of the other possible causes of slowly progressive dementia and systematically exclude those which are considered likely.

Notes

1. Tomlinson, B. E., Blessed, G., and Roth, M., Observations on the brains of non-demented old people. *J. Neurol. Sci.* 7: 331–356, 1968.
2. Tomlinson, B. E., Blessed, G., and Roth, M., Observations on the brains of demented old people. *J. Neurol. Sci.* 11: 205–242, 1970.
3. Hachinski, V. C., Lassen, N. A., and Marshall, J., Multi-infarct dementia: A cause of mental deterioration in the elderly. *Lancet* ii: 207–209, 1974.
4. Heyman, A., Therapeutic decisions in transient cerebral ischemia. *Drug Therapy*, 1979, pp. 69–75.
5. Matsuyama, H., and Nakamura, S., Senile changes in the brain in the Japanese: Incidence of Alzheimer's neurofibrillary change and senile plaques. In *Alzheimer's Disease: Senile Dementia and Related Disorders (Aging, Vol. 7)*, ed. by R. Katzman, R. D. Terry, and K. L. Bick, Raven Press, New York, 1978.
6. Kiloh, L. G., Pseudodementia. *Acta. Psychiat. Scand.* 37: 336–351, 1961.
7. Zung, W. W. K., A self-rating depression scale, *Arch. Gen. Psychiat.* 12: 63–70, 1965.
8. Zung, W. W. K., A rating instrument for anxiety disorders. *Psychosom.* 12: 371–379, 1971.
9. Gurland, B. J., The assessment of the mental health status of older adults. In J. E. Birren and R. Sloane (eds.), *Handbook of Mental Health and Aging*, 1979.
10. Hamilton, M., A rating scale for depression. *J. Neurol. Neurosurg. Psychiat.* 23: 56–62, 1960.
11. Sternberg, D. E., and Jarvik, M. E., Memory functions in depression: Improvement with antidepressant medication. *Arch. Gen. Psychiat.* 33: 219–224, 1976.
12. Wells, C. E., Pseudodementia. *Amer. J. Psychiat.* 136: 895–900, 1979.
13. Ashford, W., and Ford, C. V., Use of MAO inhibitors in elderly patients. *Am. J. Psychiat.* 136:11, 1466–1467, 1979.
14. Hoehn, M. M., and Yahr, M. D., Parkinsonism: Onset, progression and mortality. *Neurology* (Minneapolis) 17: 427–442, 1967.

15. Merritt, H. H., *A Textbook of Neurology,* 5th ed., Lea & Febiger, Philadelphia, 1973, pp. 462–471.

16. Pollack, M., and Hornabrook, R. W., The prevalence, natural history, and dementia of Parkinson's disease. *Brain* 89: 429–448, 1966.

17. Selby, G., Parkinson's disease. In P. J. Vinken and G. W. Bruyn (eds.), *Handbook of Clinical Neurology,* Vol. 6, North-Holland, Amsterdam, 1968, pp. 173–211.

18. Loranger, A. W., Goodell, H., and McDowell, F., Intellectual impairment in Parkinson's syndrome. *Brain* 95: 402–412, 1972.

19. Martin, W. E., Loewenson, R. B., and Resch, J. A., Parkinson's disease: Clinical analysis of 100 patients. *Neurology* (Minneapolis) 23: 783–790, 1973.

20. Sweet, R. D., McDowell, H., and Fergenson, J. S., Mental symptoms in Parkinson's disease during treatment with levodopa. *Neurology* (Minneapolis) 26: 305–310, 1976.

21. Diamond, S. G., Markham, C. H., and Treciokas, L. J., Long term experience with L-dopa: Efficacy, progression and mortality. In W. Birkmayer and O. Hornykiewicz (eds.), *Advances in Parkinsonism,* Roche, Basel, 1976, pp. 444–455.

22. Lieberman, A., Dziatolowski, M., Kupersmith, M., Serby, M., and Goldstein, M., Dementia in Parkinson disease, *Ann. Neurol.* 6: 355–359, 1979.

23. Hakim, A. M., and Mathieson, G., Basis of dementia in Parkinson's disease. *Lancet* ii: 729, 1978.

24. Hakim, A. M., and Mathieson, G., Dementia in Parkinson disease: A neuropathologic study. *Neurology* 29: 1209–1214, 1979.

25. Pomara, N., Reisberg, B., Albers, S., Ferris, S., and Gershon, S., Incidence of extrapyramidal symptoms in patients with mild to moderate age-related cognitive impairment. Unpublished manuscript.

26. Forno, L. S., and Alvord, E. C., Jr., The pathology of parkinsonism. In F. H. McDowell and C. H. Markham (eds.), *Recent Advances in Parkinson's Disease,* F. A. Davis Company, Philadelphia, 1971, Chap. 5.

27. Rosenblum, W. I., and Ghatak, N. R., Lewy bodies in the presence of Alzheimer's disease. *Arch. Neurol.* 36: 170–171, 1979.

28. Woodard, J. C., Concentric hyaline inclusion body formation in mental disease: Analysis of 27 cases. *J. Neuropath. Exp. Neurol.* 21: 442–449, 1962.

29. Hakim, S., and Adams, R. D., The special clinical problem of symptomatic hydrocephalus with normal cerebrospinal fluid pressure: Observations on cerebrospinal fluid hydrodynamics. *J. Neurol. Sci.* 2: 307–327, 1965.

30. Roberts, M. A., and Caird, F. I., Computerized tomography and in-

tellectual impairment in the elderly. *J. Neurol. Neurosurg. Psychiat.* 39: 986–989, 1976.

31. Fox, J. H., Kaszniak, A. W., and Huckman, M., Computerized tomographic scanning not very helpful in dementia—nor in craniopharyngiomia. *New England J. Med.* 300: 437, 1979.

32. Claveria, L. E., Moseley, J. F., and Stevenson, J. F., The clinical significance of "cerebral atrophy" as shown by CAT. In G. H. du Boulay and I. F. Moseley (eds.), *First European Seminar on Computerized Tomography in Clinical Practice,* Springer-Verlag, Berlin, 1977, pp. 213–217.

33. deLeon, M. J., Ferris, S. H., Blau, I., George, A. E., Reisberg, B., Kricheff, I. I., and Gershon, S., Correlations between computerized tomographic changes and behavioral deficits in senile dementia. *Lancet* ii: 859, 1979.

34. de Leon, M. J., Ferris, S. H., George, A. E., Reisberg, B., Kricheff, I. I., and Gershon, S., Computed tomography evaluations of brain-behavior relationships in senile dementia of the Alzheimer's type. *Neurobiology of Aging, Experimental and Clinical Research,* Vol. 1, No. 1, 69–79, 1980.

35. Reisberg, B., de Leon, M. J., Ferris, S. H., George, A. E., Reiser, M., and Gershon, S. Psychiatric assessments of cognitive impairment and brain changes in senile dementia. Presented at the American Geriatric Society, April 16–18, 1980, Chicago.

36. Adams, R. D., Fisher, G. M., Hakim, S., Ojemann, R. G., and Sweet, W. H., Symptomatic occult hydrocephalus with "normal" cerebrospinal-fluid pressure, *New England J. Med.* 273: 117–126, 1965.

37. Marsden, C. D., and Harrison, M. J. G., Correspondence: Presenile dementia. *Brit. Med. J.* 3: 50–51, 1972.

38. Jellinger, K., Neuropathological aspects of dementias resulting from abnormal blood and cerebrospinal fluid dynamics. *Acta Neurol. Belg.* 76: 83–102, 1976.

39. Katzman, R., Normal pressure hydrocephalus. In *Alzheimer's Disease: Senile Dementia and Related Disorders (Aging,* Vol. 7), ed. by R. Katzman, R. D. Terry, and K. L. Bick, Raven Press, New York, 1978, pp. 115–124.

40. Katzman, R., Normal pressure hydrocephalus. In *Dementia,* ed. by C. E. Wells, Davis, Philadelphia, 1977, pp. 69–92.

41. Illingworth, R. D., Logue, V., Symon, L., and Uemura, K., The ventriculocaval shunt in the treatment of adult hydrocephalus: Results and complications in 101 patients. *J. Neurosurg.* 35: 681–685, 1971.

42. Wood, J. H., Bartlet, D., James, A. E., Jr., and Udvarhelyi, G. B., Normal pressure hydrocephalus: Diagnosis and patient selection for shunt surgery. *Neurology* (Minneapolis) 24: 517–526, 1974.

43. Stein, S. C., and Langfitt, T. W., Normal-pressure hydrocephalus: Predicting the results of cerebrospinal fluid shunting. *J. Neurosurg.* 41: 463–470, 1974.

44. Fann, W. E., and Wheless, J. C., Therapeutic principles in the management of movement disorders in elderly patients. *Interdisciplinary Topics in Gerontology,* Vol. 15, Karger, Basel, 1979, pp. 194–210.

Chapter 5

The Evolution of Senility

SENILITY IS A VERY GRADUAL PROCESS. In medical terminology it follows an "insidious" course. That is to say, an exceedingly serious and even life-threatening condition may develop very gradually and almost imperceptibly from seemingly innocuous beginnings.

Three distinct phases can be recognized. The earliest phase may be called "forgetfulness." During this stage deficits develop which are evident to the victim and, frequently, to the spouse. The deficit is not particularly evident to more casual observers, however, and is entirely invisible to a stranger. Even sophisticated psychometric tests may fail to elicit definite evidence of deficit at this early stage. Similarly, an experienced psychiatrist knowledgeable in geriatrics can often detect only "subjective" deficits at this early stage. That is to say, the psychiatric interviewer can only elicit deficits which the victim is willing to confess. Without the candid cooperation of the person whose memory is "not quite what it used to be," even an experienced clinical interviewer cannot identify deficit with any assurance at this time.

The process of forgetfulness begins in a very similar fashion for most people. The earliest deficits are almost invariably not being able to remember names and forgetting where one has placed objects. The name-finding deficit generally begins with a person's finding increased difficulty thinking of the name of an individual or a place that was formerly quite familiar. For example, an insurance salesman who formerly had rapid recall of the names of literally hundreds of his clients and associates may find that he is now able to remember the names of only his best customers and more intimate colleagues. To the salesman there is a definite, clearly evident decrement in his formerly impressive memory powers. Nevertheless, to his associates he is essentially the same. He can still conduct business as successfully as previously, even though he may have to avoid using the client's name in the course of a sales presentation. Even more importantly, he is still the same person; that is to say, his personality remains essentially the same as it always has been.

Interestingly, at the very beginning, when the forgetfulness phase is most mild, individuals are able to remember the names of new people to whom they are introduced as well (or as poorly) as formerly. It is specifically names of persons and things which once were stored away somewhere in their brains that they are no longer able to recall. At a somewhat later point in the evolution of the forgetfulness phase, however, individuals do begin to have difficulty remembering names of things which may be new to them as well.

As mentioned, the other frequently encountered problem in the forgetfulness phase is forgetting where objects have been placed. This is usually only a minor annoyance. People may forget where they put their keys, or begin searching for a card which they thought they had placed in a drawer.

These early deficits in remembering names and remembering where objects have been placed are strikingly similar to the kinds of memory deficits which are observed in certain other psychological conditions. Resemblance to the kinds of memory deficits observed in anxiety states is the most striking case of this. Anxiety is a universal human phenomenon; all of us have experienced being anxious. Whereas a certain level of anxiety is stimulating and may improve our thinking and performance, high levels of anxiety definitely interfere with our thinking (cognitive) processes. All of us have had the experience of being anxious and having difficulty recalling persons, places, and other stored-away information which we would ordinarily be able to retrieve from our memories. Similarly, we often experience difficulty locating objects when we are anxious. Increased anxiety is associated with concentration difficulties. When we are anxious, we find that we may have to read a paragraph over and over before it will "sink in"; in other words, we experience difficulty with learning acquisition. Also, we may start to say something and "lose track" of what it was we were saying, a sign of poor concentration. These kinds of deficits in acquiring new material and in concentrating are very similar to the kinds of problems experienced during the latter part of the forgetfulness stage.

Nevertheless, despite the similarity between the cognitive deficits observed in anxiety and those found during the phase of forgetfulness, anxiety itself is generally not a significant component of this phase. The usual response to the memory problems experienced in the forgetfulness phase is appropriate concern and productive countermeasures so as to minimize the impact of the newly found decrement in intellectual ability. Since anxiety is not manifest, anxiety itself cannot explain the deficits encountered in forgetfulness.

How, then, can we explain the astounding similarity between the memory deficits seen in anxiety and those experienced in early senility? Is there a common process encountered in many different types of memory impairment? The answer to the latter question clearly is "no." The cognitive deficits observed in anxiety and in forgetfulness are decidedly different from those observed in many other conditions associated with memory loss. For example, psychiatrists are familiar with memory problems encountered shortly after electroconvulsive treatments (ECT). These treatments are known to be useful in the amelioration of certain very severe kinds of depressive illness. The treatments consist of passing an electric current through the brain so as to produce a seizure identical to the kind of seizure which occurs in certain forms of epilepsy. The memory deficit observed after these ECT treatments is somewhat different from the condition we have described accompanying anxiety and forgetfulness. After ECT, the patient shows the greatest deficit in recalling events from the past. Post-ECT events may be recalled more readily. For example, an elderly patient whom I treated for a severe depression asked me, "What am I doing here, doctor? How did I get here?" When I asked him to recall the events of that day and tested his concentration by having him do serial subtractions out loud, his recall was relatively good.

Psychosis, epilepsy, and head trauma are other conditions in which a form of amnesia is encountered that can be distinguished from the kinds of cognitive deficits seen in anxiety and in forgetfulness. For example, after an acute psychotic episode, during which a person may have visions which those around him cannot see, hear voices which are inaudible to others or have fixed, patently false beliefs which psychiatrists term "delusions," frequently an amnesia occurs for the entire experience. If a psychiatrist subsequently queries a patient on what happened, what the patient experienced and thought, he often discovers that the psychotic episode has been forgotten.

Similarly, a "postictal" amnesia characteristically occurs after a grand mal epileptic seizure. There is complete loss of recall for events prior to and during the seizure. After the seizure the victim usually falls asleep. When the victim awakens, there is no memory whatsoever of the convulsion or of events immediately preceding it; in other respects, however, memory has returned to normal.

An epileptic never recalls events during the so-called "ictal" or "dreamlike" state which precedes a seizure or during the seizure itself. Hence even people who have had dozens of seizures can only describe what others have told them occurred during the seizures; they have no personal recollection of the events. Other aspects of memory and thinking processes of most epileptics remain intact.

Conditions called "anterograde" and "retrograde" amnesia for events occurring, respectively, following and preceding a head concussion are also known to occur. Once again, the syndrome has characteristic aspects. The retrograde amnesia after a blow to the head generally does not extend beyond a period of one week. Anterograde amnesia disappears slowly. Frequently, memory is never completely restored for the postconcussional amnesic period.[1]

Recent experiments have begun to reveal the chemical mechanisms which form the basis of many types of memory loss. For example, the amnesias produced by electroconvulsive shock and convulsive drugs could be the consequence of the seizures which they produce. This has been shown not to be the case because direct electrical stimulation of specific brain regions—below the level necessary to produce seizures—also produces amnesia in some cases.[2,3] Other experiments have shown that injections of adrenal hormone* can produce amnesia for past experiences and events (retrograde amnesia).[4] If we give a certain chemical called PB2** prior to the administration of adrenalin, we can block the production of amnesia. This is really not so surprising, since PB2 is a known adrenalin-blocking drug. What is surprising, however, is the finding that PB2 reduced retrograde amnesias pro-

---

* Specifically, adrenalin (epinephrine) or adrenocorticotrophic hormone (ACTH).
** PB2 is phenoxybenzamine, an α-adrenergic blocking agent.

duced by many other causes. For example, PB2 injected before learning prevented amnesia produced by a chemical which blocks protein synthesis. PB2 also prevented amnesia produced by electrical stimulation of the brain. Also, PB2 prevented amnesia which would ordinarily occur after the administration of a chemical convulsant agent. These findings indicate that a single chemical mechanism can block retrograde amnesia produced in many different ways.[5] They seem to provide strong evidence for similar chemical processes underlying the development of many different kinds of memory loss.

We can now return to the question posed earlier—namely, how can we explain the similarity between the memory deficits seen in persons with anxiety and those observed in early senility?

We know that anxiety causes changes in body chemistry and in brain chemistry. We have also seen that certain kinds of changes in brain chemicals are consistently seen in senility. For example, we have described the consistent finding of a decrease in acetylcholine in certain areas of the brain compared with other neurotransmitter chemicals. Logically, we can hypothesize that the chemical basis for the memory loss found in anxiety and that observed in early senility may be similar, if not identical.

One of the most popular modern myths surrounding the development of senility is the "if you don't use it, you lose it" myth. This popular belief holds that senility often begins to develop, or that people become forgetful, when they stop exercising their minds with stimulating thoughts and ideas. It is essentially an optimistic belief. "If one only remains active in body and in mind, everything will be okay."

This popular belief has recently received some support in medical circles. Dr. James Folsom, a psychiatrist who is currently the director of the well-known ICD Rehabilitation and Research Center in New York City, has developed a humanistic form of therapy based upon this belief which he calls Reality Orientation. Dr. Folsom has been quoted as stating, "I don't believe in 'senility'—what is frequently called 'senility' is actually a dehumanization and depersonalization that is inflicted on people led to believe all their lives that the old get 'senile'—and so they become ready victims when presented with such problems as loss of spouse or job, retirement, lessened ability to work, a stroke or heart attack."[6]

These are strong and optimistic words, but are they based on any scientific reality? In many ways this is a "chicken and the egg" issue. Do people retire because they develop brain failure, or do people develop brain failure because they retire? Fortunately, there is an empirical* answer which is easily arrived at by studying the forgetfulness stage. We have stated that the disability during this early stage is not so severe as to prevent persons from continuing their former activities, although their performance may be somewhat impaired. Hence we can study people during the forgetfulness stage who remain active and involved in work and recreation, and can see if their activities prevent the development of senility. Some of our patients at the Geriatric Study and Treatment Program at the N.Y.U. Medical Center provide striking refutations of Dr. Folsom's statement and the popular myth which it perpetrates.

The example of one of our patients, a physician whom we will call Werner L., demonstrates the inaccuracy of the "active body, active mind" theory.

Dr. Werner L. is currently chairman of a major medical department. He was referred to us by a physician friend familiar with his current difficulties and with our work. Our testing confirmed what was painfully obvious to him: his memory was slipping. He remains as active and involved as ever at 64 years of age. Not only does he run a large medical department within a medical school, but he continues to teach and to publish scholarly research. My own interviews confirm that he reads prolifically. He follows the medical literature, also reads popular literature, and keeps abreast of current events. His knowledge and scholarship remain impressive. We once discussed an article which we had both happened to read months before in a state medical society journal. The article was on the life of the first American Indian female physician. He and I were equally impressed with the woman's fortitude and accomplishments. His memory of the article appeared better than mine.

Despite these continuing activities, Dr. L. is showing unmistakable signs of the forgetfulness phase. His memory for names was formerly every bit as impressive as his memory in other areas. Dr. L. currently has five secretaries. They are the same five whom he had last year, but he cannot remember their names. When he gives a talk at a medical conference, he now has to talk around the names of diseases and phenomena which he has known and spoken of for decades. His

---

* "Empirical" is the scientist's word for "derived from . . . experience or experiment," or "depending upon experience or observation alone, without using . . . theory." C. L. Burnhart and Stein (eds.), *The American College Dictionary*, New York, 1961, p. 394.

developing problems are painfully obvious to him and to his wife. His ability to retain his job, which he loves dearly, is dependent upon his ability to conceal his deficit from his peers. This he has done, until now, successfully.

Werner L. was born in Germany. He was raised in the Protestant faith, to which his formerly Jewish mother had converted many years before he was born. He had an older brother who became a physician. Werner followed in his brother's footsteps and also set out to become a physician.

Werner's childhood interests focused upon medicine and science, and he remained uninvolved in politics during the period in which the Nazis rose to power in Germany. He succeeded in gaining admission to a German medical school. He enrolled and diligently pursued his medical studies. Gradually, however, events intruded that disrupted his political complacency. Two of his professors, a husband and wife who were both Jewish physicians, committed suicide. Their bodies were brought into the emergency room while a friend was serving as a clerk there. Rumors abounded.

Werner was in medical school on the famous "crystal night" of October 1938, the night when the Nazis, already in firm control of Germany, rampaged through the streets destroying the windows of shops and property known to be Jewish-owned. When the Nazis learned of his family's partially Jewish ancestry, he was dismissed from medical school and his brother was forced to give up his job. One day the Nazis issued a proclamation that resulted in the seizure of all persons whom they defined as Jews between 16 and 60. He and his brother were sent to Auschwitz. His father, 61 years of age, was permitted to remain at home.

Werner's brother had done a research elective in a Swiss medical school several years before. While there he became good friends with a woman, Helga, who worked in the bacteriology department. They remained friends for years afterwards. Werner's father, aware of the friendship, wrote to Helga about his children's plight. She agreed to help. His father mailed Helga the German passports for Werner and his brother. Helga took the passports to the Canadian embassy and pleaded for visas. She was refused. Helga returned to the embassy daily for a week, pleading and finally crying for her friends. The officials were moved. They stamped visas on the passports. Helga sent the passports back to Werner's father. He immediately went to the Gestapo with the documents.

In the interim Werner and his brother had been living in barracks in Auschwitz. They were provided only with flimsy summer concentration camp outfits, nothing more. Winter came. Many of the inmates died from exposure to the freezing weather. The Nazis believed in regimentation. They continually gave orders and marched the inmates back and forth. Those who could not tolerate the discipline or who became ill were executed or died. All the inmates became emaciated from the meager rations permitted them.

The passports for Werner and his brother arrived, and they were called from the barracks by the authorities. The Nazis would not permit anyone who showed scars or signs of possible mistreatment to leave the concentration camps. Werner and his brother were forced to undress and pass inspection before they could leave the camp. His brother had an infection around the nail of his index finger which he was able to conceal successfully by tucking his fingers into his palm. They passed. They were released.

Werner and his brother returned to Germany and went to Switzerland with their passports. Werner was emaciated. His hair had grayed. His mind, apparently, remained brilliant. He enrolled in medical school and completed his studies in Switzerland. Years later he emigrated to the United States, where he learned English, passed the necessary medical qualifications for licensing, completed specialty training to meet American requirements, and rose to become a department chairman. His memory remained excellent, his intellectual prowess formidable.

In Werner's words, "I do not fear old age because I have known hardship early in life." The "dehumanization and depersonalization" inflicted upon Werner and his brother by the Nazis appear to have left their mental prowess intact. The physical abuse, the emotional upheaval, the personal humiliation, even when combined to yield a horror difficult to contemplate, clearly did not result in irrevocable mental senescence. Werner did not become forgetful as a result of his experiences in Europe. He retained the cognitive capacity to attain an enviable professional standing in a foreign land, with an unfamiliar tongue, in an intellectually demanding field.

How then do we explain his current forgetfulness? Surely not by "a dehumanization and depersonalization inflicted on old people led to believe all their lives that the old get 'senile' . . . ." Senility is not a religion. Believing all one's life that the old get senile will not make it so. Senility is not wish fulfillment. Neither is senility the antithesis of wish fulfillment. It may be a condition which we fear, but it is not the result of our fears. Nor would a lack of "mental exercise" seem to be a plausible causative factor in this accomplished, erudite man who continues to read prolifically as well as to function as an administrator, clinician, teacher, and scholar.

In the preceding chapters we have described in some detail the physical and chemical changes in the brain which accompany the senile process. These very real alterations in the substance of the brain certainly find expression in observable changes in emotion and behavior. Conversely, an individual's emotional reactions to the real brain changes which are occurring will certainly help to determine the extent of the disability. However, although emotional and behavioral changes are inevitably *associated with* any condition such as senility, which profoundly affects the brain, these emotional and behavioral changes certainly are not the *cause* of the condition.

Viral or bacterial infectious agents often result in fevers which can affect the brain in many ways. In their mildest form the effects become manifest behaviorally as fatigue and irritability. More severe behavioral manifestations of fevers include delerious states with disorientation and confusion. However, physicians and laymen alike currently recognize that these emotional states (with rare exceptions) are not the *cause* of fever, but rather the *result* of a condition brought on by an infectious agent. Analogously, a brain tumor will produce cognitive and personality changes, with anxiety and ultimately "dehumanization." Clearly, this does not mean that personality factors, fears, or dehumanization causes brain tumors.

Senility is similar to febrile illness (fever) and cerebral neoplasm (brain tumor) in that it affects the brain profoundly and the consequences of the effects are changes in emotions and thinking process. Before the great discoveries of modern times in the area of infectious disease, many fevers and deleriums were indeed believed to be caused by "bewitching" and similar "psychological" mechanisms. Brain cancers also were frequently attributed to behavioral processes before much became known about these devastating conditions. Although the causes of senility are not currently as clearly identified as those of many fevers and tumors, the underlying causes of senility are undoubtedly also largely independent of emotional processes.

The second identifiable stage in the evolution of senility may be referred to as "the confused phase." In this phase the thinking deficit becomes more obvious, particularly to those who have known the vic-

tim previously. Unlike the "forgetful" person, who recognizes an incipient deficit and is most frequently appropriately concerned about it,
for the "confused" person the magnitude and implications of the
deficit become too painful for conscious recognition. As with any major
illness or loss, the dominant response is one of denial. When the confused individual is confronted with a challenging situation that cannot
be avoided or denied, overt anxiety develops. Many confused persons
successfully evade anxiety by a combination of withdrawal from stress-
producing activities and simultaneous denial of deficit and acceptance
of a much lower level of functioning.

The deficits in the confused phase are numerous, particularly when
one is aware of the confused person's former abilities. Initially, the major new deficits are in concentration and in recent memory. One frequent manifestation is people's repeating themselves during the course
of a conversation. When this becomes overt, psychiatrists refer to it as
"rambling" or "perseveration" or some other specific form of what is
known as "loosening of associations."

Subjectively, these concentration and recent memory problems
may become manifest even before they become evident to observers.
Frequently, people with these deficits recognize that they have no
sooner finished reading an article than they have forgotten what they
have just read. Some complain of concentration problems and having
to read a passage over and over. Many patients have described having
read a book from cover to cover and having completely forgotten what
it was about.

Another deficit frequently experienced early in the confused phase
is in remembering appointments. Initially, this problem is correctable
by simply keeping an appointment book and recording all future
engagements. Later on, confused-phase people find they have to refer
to their book constantly and often still require additional assistance—
for instance, their spouses may nevertheless have to remind them further of their schedules.

Addresses and telephone numbers which once were familiar are
often recalled by confused-phase individuals only with difficulty. They
may, for example, forget their children's addresses even though their
offspring have not moved for years and they formerly knew their addresses well.

Problems with names assume embarrassing proportions. Confused
persons frequently can recall the names of only some of their grand-

children. Later on they begin to confuse the names of their children and their grandchildren.

Early in the confused phase people virtually always subjectively feel and complain that their memory of recent things has suffered more than their memory of the past. Objective relative weighting of these two kinds of memory impairment is difficult to achieve. For example, a clinician may observe that a confused person does not recall the name or the contents of a movie he or she saw the previous evening. The person may also fail to recall the name of a childhood friend known for many years.

Difficulty with traveling and with orientation also becomes manifest during this stage. Often our confused patients who continue to travel on their own to our clinic are delayed for their appointments because they have forgotten to get off the bus at the proper time, or because they started to walk in the wrong direction when they emerged from the train station. These same people frequently have difficulty recalling the date and the day of the week. Sometimes they will know the day and the month, but be inaccurate when asked the year.

Mrs. Adams is a confused-phase patient in our program. Occasionally she comes to the Millhauser Laboratories by herself, and on other occasions her husband accompanies her. Mrs. Adams is an attorney. She states that she is semiretired but that she still maintains an active part-time legal practice in association with her husband, also an attorney. She denies experiencing anything more than minor memory problems. "Otherwise, I couldn't work as an attorney. I couldn't go to court. I couldn't prepare a case."

Her explanation seems perfectly logical unless a clinician "tests" her memory and her intellectual abilities. Although Mrs. Adams is an attorney, she has difficulty recalling the name of the state governor. Similarly she knows the President and the Vice President, but couldn't recall the previous President.

"I'm not interested in current events and I'm terrible with names," she explains. Once again her explanation seems plausible but somewhat unlikely.

"What is your religion?"
"Catholic."
"Do you go to church?"
"Sometimes."

"Who is the Pope?"

"Pope John."

"What nationality is he?"

"Italian."

"What nationality are you?"

"Polish."

"We have a Polish Pope now. Do you know who he is?"

"That's right."

"Who is he?"

"I can't think of his name."

"What's going on in the world?"

"Nothing special. The usual wars and things."

"Oh, really. Where are they fighting?"

"No place special."

"You're a lawyer. What kind of law do you practice?"

"General practice."

"What kind of cases do you handle?"

"Divorce, things like that."

"Where did you go to law school?"

"Columbia."

"And where did you do a clerkship?"

"They didn't have clerkships in those days."

"Oh. What was your first job then?"

"I don't know. It was a long time ago, but soon afterwards I got married and went into practice with my husband."

Like many confused persons, Mrs. Adams seemed to have what psychiatrists call a "flattening of affect." By this we mean that there appeared to be a decrease in her emotional responsiveness. Certainly this includes an absence of vivaciousness and joie de vivre. Laymen would describe Mrs. Adams as "not very lively."

Frequently, relatives or inexperienced health professionals mistake this lack of emotion for depression. But it is not depression. If one asks the patients if they are unhappy, the answer is "No," "Not really," or "I don't think so." Similarly there is no hopelessness or despair. Nor do these people feel that life is anything other than worthwhile. They decidedly wish to continue living despite their problems.

For a former Columbia Law School graduate, Mrs. Adams's memory would not seem to be very good. But how bad is it really? More specifically, how much have her memory and her thinking abilities deteriorated? It is difficult to get a satisfactory answer to this important question simply by interviewing Mrs. Adams. Psychological testing can help somewhat. We know that a person's vocabulary tends to be relatively well preserved in comparison with other aspects of thinking ability and knowledge. Hence Mrs. Adams's vocabulary test score may remain in the near excellent range whereas her scores in other areas may be far below what one would expect of a woman with her intelligence.

Clinically, the most accurate way to assess Mrs. Adams's apparent deficit is to interview her in her husband's presence. Mr. Adams's responses give the story a very different flavor.

"She doesn't really have clients anymore," he explains. "I let her come to the office, but she hasn't tried a case in years. She's completely disorganized. She keeps misplacing and losing documents. But I'd rather have her at the office. It makes her feel better. She's always worked, she wouldn't know what to do at home.

"She used to be very interested in politics and current events. She read *Newsweek* regularly and the *Times* almost daily. We were involved in politics at one time. In fact, we were talking about the governor only yesterday."

"Mrs. Adams, who is the Pope?"
"Pope John."
"What nationality is he?"
"Italian."
"Jean, you know he's not Italian. We were watching him on TV last night. You know where he's from. Poland."
"Oh, that's right."

And so it goes. The interview of a moderately impaired confused-phase, or phase II, individual is never really complete unless a relative or friend who knows the patient well is present.

Like Mrs. Adams, many phase II individuals continue to work and even to expand the scope and richness of their lives. Unfortunately, this healthy process does not appear to defend against, or even to retard, the evolution of senility. Once again, our clinic has seen some spectacular and tragic illustrations of this truth.

Thomas was 78 years old when he came to us. After a remarkably varied career marked by continued exploration and growth, he enrolled in graduate school in his mid-fifties. He was 66 when he became a doctor of musicology. Subsequently he got his first teaching position, and in a few years his scholarship earned him the title of "professor of musicology."

I have never admired or loved any patient so much as Thomas. His face and demeanor bespoke a man whose life had been extraordinarily rich. Occasionally he would entice me with his reminiscences. But it was his present which was truly impressive. He would sit in our office reading an ancient Arabic music book, in the original classical Arabic language.

"Musicology," he explained, "is the comparative study of the musical forms of different cultures. I teach the evolution of Middle Eastern musical forms."

I suppose that helped to explain his showing up the following week with a journal of ancient Hebrew music.

It wasn't only Thomas's professional interests which appeared to be well cultivated and continuing to grow and to yield fruit. He had friends, close, personal relationships, all over the country, whom he would often set off to visit. His life and his work appeared to complement each other and to have etched their cadences upon his vigorous, ancient, lively, expressive face. His face was like that of a holy man, with a rich, full white beard merging with thick, curly, equally white hair, the two masses set off from each other by appropriately furrowed and carved features.

The tragedy was that this brilliant and wonderful man was being gradually and inexorably destroyed. He would ramble and begin to repeat himself during the course of an interview. He occasionally would turn up for an appointment at the wrong time. Although he continued to teach and to prepare lectures, he recognized that they were lacking in clarity and organization, although his knowledge remained impressive. It was a heartbreaking process to behold. After completing one of our programs, Thomas declared that he had too many things to do and therefore would be unable to resume treatment. If activity and intellectual stimulation had any relevance for the evolution of senility, Thomas would certainly have been immune to further decline. Unfortunately, his activities only served to highlight the encroaching deficits and inexorable decline.

Although denial is nearly universal in the phase II, confused condition, there are times when it is not sufficient to control underlying anxiety and the victim will seem overtly nervous. This was the case with an executive who came to our clinic at his family's recommendation, Mr.

Currin. Mr. Currin was still working and had maintained his job, but under intolerable circumstances. He was faced daily and constantly with tasks which he could not handle. His response was anxiety and inner pain. His employers took all of Mr. Currin's clients away from him and reassigned them to other officers. One day one of Mr. Currin's former clients called and asked for him by name, and he took the call. After that his boss removed the telephone from his office!

My interviews with Mr. Currin during this period revealed marked nervousness. The latter only added to his disability. Eventually, the humiliations became unbearable and Mr. Currin retired.

What a change! It was as if all of his problems had evaporated. He became calm, even overly lacking in emotion. A few weeks later he was denying any real memory problems. And in a sense he was correct. His expectations of himself and the demands of daily living had been reset at a much lower level.

The third and final phase of senility is that of "dementia." In the dementia phase the magnitude of the deficit is such as to be obvious and unquestionable, even upon only casual observation. The dementia phase may be said to begin at the point where individuals can no longer survive if left on their own. Frequently, if not watched, these people will wander off and become hopelessly lost. Indeed, many of the demented do succumb when they have gotten lost and no longer have the mental resources to save themselves. Occasionally they will freeze to death in the winter, or will starve to death in the woods.

One of our patients would wander away from her summer cottage on "walks." On a particular occasion she was gone for several hours. Her family called the police, who found her wandering aimlessly about town seven miles away from her cottage. Upon being discovered, she denied anything was wrong and insisted that she was simply going about her business. However, she had no idea where she was, had no money, had not eaten, and did not know her address.

Because of the serious problems with wandering and getting lost of our phase III persons, we strongly recommend their being provided with adequate identification. For many phase III individuals, this consists of an I.D. card or tag which they cannot pull off or which they can remove only with difficulty.

Because demented persons have lost the ability to retain virtually all new information, many of them, of necessity, begin to live in the past. One of our patients was taken to live with her son and daughter-in-law when she could no longer live on her own. Although she had lived with her children for almost a year, whenever I asked her where she lived, she gave me her former address. More strikingly, when I asked her whether she lived alone, she would answer "Yes." Could she manage on her own? Again, she would answer affirmatively. Furthermore, her son's apartment was in the same neighborhood as her former home, and if she went for a walk by herself, she invariably would return to her former home, the only one she "knew."

This lack of knowledge of the present manifests itself in other unusual ways. Some demented persons set out for work daily although they have been retired for years. One of our patients had made a movie which had been shown at the Museum of Modern Art years before. For her it was always the movie which she had worked on "last summer."

Once again, denial plays a major role in demented patients' lives. This is supplemented with other defense mechanisms against the anxiety and depression which would result from too conscious an awareness of their state. Anxiety, however, may become overt in these persons. Occasionally the anxiety finds a further outlet in aggression and hostility.

The aggression and hostility occasionally seen in demented persons is a reasonable by-product of their current circumstances, and seems to be independent of their behavior prior to the onset of their illness. One woman, who came to our clinic accompanied by a relative, had traveled more than an hour to reach us. When she arrived, she refused to be interviewed, or to "answer questions," as she put it. I convinced her to let me speak with her, and we succeeded in discussing her "feelings." As soon as we moved to any concrete topic, such as my asking her the date or the year, she became evasive, both verbally and physically, to the point of her getting up and walking out of the office. Evidently she avoided, consciously, any situations which would force her to face her limitations too directly.

Being unaware and unable to keep track of one's possessions is a painful and frightening experience. Many demented individuals respond by hiding possessions which they consider valuable. Paradoxically and irrationally, phase III persons may hide their possessions from the very persons who are responsible for them and who are assisting in keeping them alive. Subsequently, of course, when they need these treasured items, they have forgotten where they were sequestered.

Many phase III demented persons begin to experience what relatives sometimes call "illusions." These experiences take on many manifestations but generally correspond to what psychiatrists term "formal thinking disorder." More often these "illusions" initially are delusional* in nature rather than actual hallucinations.** Occasionally a demented person will insist that a dead relative is present in a room. The person frequently does not actually "see" the deceased person; however, he or she strongly *believes* the person to be right there. This frequently evolves into reveries in which the demented person will carry on one-way conversations with relatives or friends who are deceased or far away.

The title of this chapter is "The Evolution of Senility." How does senility evolve in terms of time? Does forgetfulness always, if one lives long enough, result in dementia?

We have already stated that senility is a very gradual process. Furthermore, as we know, the burgeoning scientific interest in the condition has only evolved over the past several years. The answers to many of the most important questions in this area therefore are as yet unknown. They would seem to be easily obtainable by properly designed studies extended over a sufficient period; however, the results of such studies are unavailable at present.

In the N.Y.U. Geriatric Study and Treatment Program and at a few other major research centers, preliminary information is being studied which permits us to make "educated guesses" regarding some aspects of the course and prognosis of senility.

Forgetfulness apparently does not always result in dementia. The "forgetfulness phase" may be an early manifestation of approaching Alzheimer's dementia, or it may be part of a different entity which is frequently associated with normal aging and for which the term "benign senescent forgetfulness" has been proposed. Pathologically— that is, in terms of the visible and microscopic changes occurring in the brain—benign senescent forgetfulness (BSF) may correspond to the increased loss of neuronal substance which is known to occur with age. Another likely hypothesis is that this condition is related to the low concentrations of neurofibrillary tangles which are known to occur in the brains of many so-called "normal elderly" individuals. Either or both of these conditions may evolve very slowly, or they may even remain stationary and not worsen for a considerable period of time.

The brain is a plastic organ. If it is damaged in certain areas, other

---

* A delusion is a fixed, false belief which is maintained contrary to both logic and reality.

** A hallucination is a subjective sensory experience which other persons in the environment cannot experience. For example, a person has a "vision" which other people cannot see or hears a voice which other people cannot hear.

areas of the brain will very gradually take over the function which may originally have been entirely destroyed. Strokes provide a very dramatic example of the brain's resilience. After a stroke, or "cerebral infarction," which is another name for the same condition, parts of the brain are destroyed completely and other areas severely injured. The result of the event is frequently loss of speech and paralysis. However, unless another insult to the brain occurs, people gradually recover from these devastating conditions. Indeed, years later some people may dramatically recover and be capable of walking and speaking again.

Similarly, the brain may gradually adjust to the age-related changes which underlie the development of BSF. What this implies is that some forgetful people may not necessarily get worse with time, and indeed may actually improve! Preliminary results obtained from our center do indeed indicate that some forgetful persons appear to improve in their thinking abilities over the course of one to two years rather than get worse, as one might expect.

In the opening chapters we described the brain changes which occur in Alzheimer's disease, the major cause of senile dementia. It will be recalled that Alzheimer's disease does not ordinarily occur in animals other than human beings. Other kinds of age-related changes in learning and thinking abilities have been shown, however, to occur in aging animals. Specifically, aging animals tend to forget new material which they have learned more quickly than young animals. Also, aging animals learn somewhat more slowly than younger ones. These kinds of deficits are very similar to those experienced by elderly persons during the forgetful phase who forget where they have placed things or forget names they formerly knew.

Hence animal studies would definitely support our belief that phase I is often a relatively benign, age-related condition which is associated with certain kinds of brain changes but which does not necessarily progress to Alzheimer's disease and the resulting severe dementia. Indeed, it appears that some phase I individuals actually improve as time goes on.

Individuals who have entered the second, confused phase probably are showing early signs of more serious illness. In most cases properly diagnosed phase II persons probably do have early Alzheimer's disease. For these persons, as well as for the more severe phase III dements, the progression, although inexorable, varies considerably. Some people may go from phase I to phase III in a year; others may show equivalent changes over the course of a decade. For phase III persons life expectancy is definitely decreased because of the lessened ability of these persons to care for themselves. Nevertheless, even phase III demented persons may live for many years if they are adequately supported and cared for.

If the condition is so variable, if Alzheimer's disease can proceed so rapidly or so slowly, then it may be possible for scientists to learn the mechanism which determines the speed of Alzheimer's changes. If they can discover this secret, then perhaps scientists can alter the mechanisms to their own ends and retard, or possibly even stop, the progress of Alzheimer's disease. These hopes and speculations lead us to the subject of the treatment of senility, its realities and its future.

Before discussing treatment, however, we will need a clearer picture of the total process. We need to understand what happens when a normal intelligent person becomes increasingly forgetful, then subsequently becomes confused, and ultimately becomes demented. We need to understand in finer detail how these processes affect the lives of the victims and those who love them. A better comprehension of these changes should enable us to focus more directly upon potential intervention strategies.

Notes

1. Nemiah, J. C., Hysterical neuroses, dissociative type. In *Comprehensive Textbook of Psychiatry/II*, ed. by A. M. Freedman, H. I. Kaplan, and B. J. Sadock, Williams & Wilkins Company, Baltimore, 1975, pp. 1220-1231.
2. Gold, P. E., Zornetzer, S. F., and McGaugh, J. L. In G. Newton and A. Riesen (eds.), *Advances in Psychobiology*, Vol. 2, Wiley-Interscience, New York, 1974, pp. 64-75.
3. McGaugh, J. L., and Gold, P. E. In M. R. Rosenzweig and E. L. Bennett, (eds.), *Neural Mechanisms of Learning and Memory*, M.I.T. Press, Cambridge, Mass., 1976, pp. 549-560.
4. Gold, P. E., van Buskirk, R., and Haycock, J. W., Effects of posttraining epinephrine injections on retention of avoidance training in mice, *Behav. Biol.* 20: 197, 1977.
5. Paul, E., Gold, P. E., and Sternberg, D. B., Retrograde amnesia produced by several treatments: Evidence for a common neurobiological mechanism. *Science* 201: 367-369, 1978.
6. Quoted in Arthur S. Freese, *The End of Senility*, Arbor House, New York, 1978, p. 151.

Chapter 6

Joe: A Case of Senility

A REAL UNDERSTANDING OF SENILITY can be gained only by understanding how the process gradually and irrevocably alters the lives of those whom it afflicts. The process, of course, varies somewhat in different individuals. No mixture or distillate of evolutionary processes can provide a genuine understanding. We shall follow the more accurate "empirical" approach and tell the tale of one man, Joe, as observed by his loving and devoted spouse, Ilia.

Joe S. was a successful newspaperman. He was known for his ability to research a complex and socially important story and to put the information together in such a way that the general public could readily grasp its importance. One of his most memorable contributions from a medical standpoint was an article on the hazards of cigarette smoking which appeared in a national periodical in the 50s. The article synthesized the medical findings regarding the personal health dangers of cigarettes and created a public climate which made the subsequent historic Surgeon General's report more believable and, perhaps, more palatable.

Joe spent the last 20 years of his 43-year career reporting from the United Nations. He had an enviable memory. He would listen to a speech, return to his office, and dictate a story. He did this virtually without notes. He used notes only to confirm a date or the spelling of a person's name. When the newspaper he worked for ceased publication, Joe was ultimately forced to retire. Subsequently he remained active by freelancing articles for magazines.

Joe was 68 at the time of his enforced retirement. His wife and he had been together more than 40 years. She remained his lover, companion, and assistant. Ilia, as always, continued to type out the stories which Joe had dictated. She knew his abilities and style better than anyone. Shortly after Joe's retirement, at the time when he was freelancing stories for magazines, Ilia became aware of a change in Joe's previously enviable performance. His dictations began to lose their customary flow. Joe would hesitate and stop to look up a fact or a name. He seemed to encounter some difficulty finding exactly the proper word for what he wished to say. He also appeared to forget what it was he had started to say and was forced to return to his references to enable him to recapture his thought.

However, the quality of Joe's finished work retained its excellence. He wrote a story at about this time on workmen's compensation benefits. The story was so well received that Joe received a large bonus over and above the amount contractually owed him. But the former facility with which the story would have been written was noticeably, if only to himself and to Ilia, diminished.

Joe was understandably disturbed by his "loss of memory." It was he who saw the newspaper advertisement for our memory program at the Millhauser Laboratories of the New York University Medical Center. At the time we were investigating the value of the hyperbaric, or increased pressure, chamber for the treatment of early senility. Joe dutifully participated not only in that program but in all of our subsequent investigations over the next three years. His writings had contributed to the popular understanding of health, health policy, and medical science. Perhaps medical science could return the debt it owed him.

At the time of his initial visit to our program, Joe appeared to be in what we have termed the "forgetfulness phase" of memory decline. His distress at his loss of cognitive facility and his desire to "do something about it" are common responses at this stage. Also, the kinds of deficits which Joe was experiencing—losing the associative thread of his thoughts and having difficulty finding words—are distressingly common symptoms, particularly among the elderly. Epidemiologic studies have not been conducted, and hence we do not know and cannot even estimate how frequent these symptoms are. We do know, however, that they are increasingly common in progressively older groups of people.

In terms of the pathological brain changes discussed in the opening chapters, early Alzheimer's type changes were probably beginning to appear. Once again, the necessary investigations have not been conducted which would provide scientific evidence as to the true nature of the pathological changes accompanying the forgetfulness stage. However, it is logical to assume from what we do know about severe hippocampal brain damage and the more severe forms of cognitive impairment that neurofibrillary tangles and senile plaques were probably appearing in increased concentration on both sides of Joe's brain. These changes were probably most marked in the hippocampus but probably also located, to a lesser extent, in other brain regions, particularly the frontal and temporal cortex. The plaques and tangles, in theory, could have been observed if a technique were available for safely examining Joe's brain at this stage.

The plaques and tangles were probably not the cause of his problem, but rather a manifestation of it. Analogously, scar tissue is not the cause of an injury, but rather a visual indication that an injury has occurred.

Why these thinking problems should have begun to affect Joe at this time we do not know. Heredity probably played some role. Joe's mother was in her mid-eighties when her family came to think of her as being mentally senile. However, Joe's father lived until his late eighties apparently without ever having experienced memory decline. Undoubtedly, environmental factors also played some role in the development of Joe's condition, although the ways in which nutrition or other environmental factors interact to increase the likelihood of cognitive senescence are entirely unknown.

Many elderly people who begin to notice "forgetfulness" symptoms nearly identical to those observed by Joe and his wife seem to live with these symptoms for many years without any further decline. Joe, as we shall see, was not so fortunate.

That summer Ilia and Joe used the money which they had received from the workmen's compensation article to finance a trip to Japan. Joe had turned 69. For practical purposes he and Ilia remained in good health, and it appeared an ideal time for a trip abroad.

The closeness and the demands of the trip highlighted new deficits which had not been apparent previously. It was at approximately this time that Joe began to manifest symptoms of what we have termed the "confused phase." Ilia observed that Joe would have to inquire several times regarding the schedule for the day. He couldn't seem to keep in mind what time the bus was departing. During tours Joe would ask the guide questions about topics which had been discussed only a few minutes before. When the party went to a restaurant, Joe frequently had difficulty finding his way back to their table after a trip to the lavatory. Ilia, forever vigilant, would wave to him, signaling their location. Once, in Kyoto, this habit Joe had of losing his way became particularly noticeable when he emerged from a park lavatory and began walking off in the opposite direction, away from his group. His wife went running after him. Apparently, Joe had completely forgotten where his group had been waiting.

That autumn Joe resumed treatment at our Geriatric Study Program. He traveled 40 miles in each direction to see us, via public transportation. There were few difficulties even though Joe almost invariably came alone. He also resumed freelance work.

In November, Joe decided to visit an old friend who had recently moved. Ilia assisted by providing proper directions. Armed with the directions, Joe got into his car and left. He returned some hours later, having been unsuccessful in finding his way. It was at this point that Ilia realized that Joe was suffering from a serious problem. Until that time she and Joe merely attributed the events and lapses to "forgetfulness." Now it was evident something more was happening.

Ilia became "overprotective" as a result of these incidents. She discouraged Joe's plans for trips or errands which she felt he might no longer be able to accomplish. The changes were gradual and subtle. Ilia took upon herself a greater share of daily and household activities. Joe continued to go out on errands, if not on major journeys. The couple maintained their social contacts and activities. They continued to go to the theater, cinema, and opera together, just as they had done previously.

Over the next few years there were no dramatic changes. Joe retained his former friendliness and tolerance. There were no major personality changes. He nominally continued his semiretirement. He thought himself still actively freelancing, although no further assignments were ever actually completed. Joe appears to have been as successful as Mrs. Adams, the confused-phase attorney described in the preceding chapter, in denying the extent of his impairment at this stage. Ostensibly, "freelancing" was for Joe what daily visits to the law offices are for Mrs. Adams, an emotionally valuable but contrived "confirmation" of one's continued abilities and social worthiness. Since Joe remained personable and there were no longer any professional demands placed upon him, life went on tolerably well for him and Ilia. Joe was becoming increasingly forgetful, however. He began to forget what he had eaten and when. He would eat a dessert and subsequently ask his wife, "Honey, can I have some dessert?" When informed that he had just finished an ice cream sundae, he would camouflage his lapse of memory: "Oh yes, of course I did."

Joe had always been very neat. At 71 years of age he began to hang his clothing up peculiarly. He hung up a sports jacket with one sleeve on the hanger and the other sleeve hanging loosely. He hung up trousers before emptying his pockets, causing his change and the other contents to fall freely to the floor. The following morning he would have difficulty locating these items. In his wife's words, "It was peculiar for him. If he were slovenly, then I would understand his putting his clothes away the way he did, but he wasn't." These changes probably signaled the onset of the "dementia phase" of Joe's continuously diminishing thinking capacities.

Not long afterwards, Joe lost the ability to determine what clothing to wear. He would emerge in the morning only partially clothed or would ponder interminably the decision as to which shirt he would be wearing that day.

"I think he forgot that he had been selecting his clothes." Ilia satisfactorily solved this new problem by leaving Joe's clothing out the night before for him to put on in the morning.

At 73 Joe went into the hospital for prostatic surgery. There were no complications, and he was released shortly afterwards. It was then that living conditions at home became particularly severe. Joe appeared to have undergone a personality change as a result of his hospital experience. He would become very angry and shout and verbally attack people without apparent provocation.

The hospital experience may have contributed to this change in his behavior. During his brief hospitalization at an excellent private facility, Joe was frequently placed in restraints. Leather bands were tied around his wrists and ankles to prevent him from wandering off or falling out of bed. Although Ilia arranged for around-the-clock special nursing care, even the private nurses felt obligated to employ the restraints at certain times, such as when they had to leave temporarily to go for dinner. As a result of these experiences, if the nurses went to hold Joe's wrist to take his pulse, Joe feared that he was being restrained, and he would become very angry.

When Joe came home from the hospital, he was impossible to live with. He was unable to sit still. He would get up from a chair and then sit down again repeatedly. He continually went to the door to leave his apartment. He would unfasten the locks and walk into the hall. If Ilia had not been constantly alert, he would have wandered out onto the city streets and undoubtedly would have gotten hopelessly lost.

These symptoms of continuous purposeless activity are quite common in dementia-phase patients. Because no term currently exists which adequately describes the origins of such behavior, we have introduced a new term, "cognitive abulia."[1] "Abulia" is a word with Greek origins which means "loss of willpower." Cognitive abulia occurs when a patient's memory disturbance becomes so severe that the patient is unable to maintain a thought sufficiently long to complete a purposeful activity. Hence the intact energy of these dementia-phase patients is expressed as restlessness and rapidly changing, seemingly random activities. For example, when Ilia actually took Joe out onto the street, he immediately wanted to return home. Dutifully, Ilia would take him home, whereupon Joe would again insist upon leaving. Joe was like a man "possessed," wanting to do things but not really knowing what he wanted to do.

At about this time I made a home visit to determine the gravity of the situation. Ilia invited me to their home for supper. Even for a physician who spends the major portion of his time with elderly persons who have memory problems, the experience was a memorable one. Joe did not remember who I was, although we had met more than a dozen times and Ilia had explained to him repeatedly who I was and why I was invited.

Ilia made a heroic attempt to prepare a proper meal. She even went so far as to put on the table flowers and their special silver candlesticks. Each time Ilia would go into the kitchen to prepare something, Joe would wander over to the door, remove the chain, turn the lock, and make an effort to leave. Every time Joe did that, either Ilia or I would have to stop Joe at some point in the ritual and urge him to sit down. This he would do, for a minute or so, before he would set off again. Explaining to Joe that we were about to have supper and that there was no reason for him to be leaving was of no use. A few moments after the explanation and his promising to remain, he would forget what had been said and wander back to the door. I attempted to hold his attention and maintain his cooperation with conversation. How did he feel? "Fine." What had he been doing? "Nothing." What was his name? "Joe." What was his wife's name? "Like me." Had he seen his children? "Yes." When? No answer. Who were his children? No answer. Where did they live? No answer.

I inevitably tired of what was becoming a one-sided interview and returned to the more responsive Ilia. As soon as I did, Joe would resume his impatient wandering.

Despite the demands of having to watch over Joe and entertain me, Ilia eventually succeeded in putting supper on the table. The salad and the chicken were both in large bowls and we could help ourselves. Joe was unable to do this, so we served him. He seemed no longer to remember the purpose of a knife and fork. Ilia cut the chicken for him as well as served him. Otherwise his thoughts and his body would wander away from the meal. The real problem remained Joe's restlessness. He would continually forget the meal and wander away from the table. We would urge him to rejoin us, which he would, only to wander away again moments later. After seemingly endless repetitions of this process, even the saintly Ilia began to tire.

"Would you mind if I gave Joe a sleeping pill?"

"That's your decision. I can certainly see how it might be helpful," I responded, neutrally.

The tablet worked, and in half an hour she excused herself to undress Joe for bed.

"It's been like that all day," she confided upon her return. "A college girl came over for a few hours in the afternoon and took him for a walk over to the museum, but the remainder of the day I've had to spend every moment watching him. Today is the nurse's day off. I've hired a nurse for the days when I go to the office. I would lose my mind if I didn't have some time off!"

"I can certainly see your problem. It must be impossible caring for him. Have you begun to look into nursing homes?"

She began to cry. "I would feel so guilty about sending him away to a home . . . but what can I do? It's only been this way since he came home from the hospital. Do you think things will improve?"

"That would be very unlikely. A nursing home has the staff and the facilities to watch Joe and to care for him. Even a saint such as yourself couldn't continue this way. You might be in a better position to give

Joe the love he requires if you didn't have to exhaust all of your energies watching him and caring for him.''

"I just couldn't do it," she sobbed.

"Well, it can take several months finding the proper nursing home and actually finding an opening for admission to a home. Joe may get even worse. You should begin to research facilities in your area now, so that you'll be prepared when you actually make the decision.''

"For now, could you just give me something that will calm him and help him to sleep? He gets up in the middle of the night and wanders around. The other night he nearly wandered outside.''

"That would be serious. It is all the more reason for you to be considering a home. Does he have any identification?''

"I got him an I.D. necklace, but he tore it off. It bothered him.''

"You should get him a bracelet which he can't remove. I recommend having the jeweler solder the latch.

"I'll give you some sleeping pills and something to calm him, but these are only temporary solutions. Sleeping pills and sedatives become less effective after a short while, and one must continually increase the dosage. Also, they have side effects which may cause problems of their own. In the interim, you should start looking into a home.''

"Perhaps I'll begin to look. It can't hurt. The college girl has really been a help.''

"How does Joe feel about her?''

"When I first discussed it with him, he said that he didn't need anyone, that he could manage on his own.''

"Then how did you get his cooperation?''

"I told him that it would be additional company for him, and besides, he would be helping the girl by giving her a job. Also, I called up the journalism school and found someone who was interested in journalism. So, you see, I got his permission. The girl really is interested in journalism. She asks Joe questions and he enjoys it.''

"Do you know anyone, other than Joe, who has memory problems?''

"I didn't know anyone until this happened to Joe. I didn't know anything about it. At your clinic I met people with memory problems and I spoke to one man whose wife was a patient. Now I know a man, Morris. I met him and his wife, Florence, recently at a wedding. When we saw that we had a similar problem, we arranged to have brunch together. It seemed he was much worse off than Joe. He has a gradual problem which has been going on for many years. He was confused about many things, but, on the other hand, he paid for the lunch with a credit card which he took out of his wallet and which he signed for.

"Florence and I talked. We both went into the ladies' room together. We had a good cry. She has the same kind of a problem. They have a winter home in Florida. Morris loves to play golf. But already, last winter, nobody would play with him anymore because he was irrational and belligerent. So Florence hired some men to play golf with Morris. Somehow, he found out. Morris was so furious with her he nearly beat her."

"Joe appears to be sleeping soundly."

"He sleeps for a few hours, but then he sometimes gets up and wanders around. During the day he's often tired. He usually takes a nap for an hour or two."

"I would feel so guilty if I put Joe in a home." She started to sob. "He needs the care. I go to bed and put my arms around him. It's not the sex. He hasn't been interested in sex for years."

"Frequently, people with Joe's condition do lose interest in sex. However, occasionally just the opposite occurs; sometimes, in Joe's stage, they become hypersexual. This can occur for different reasons. In some cases, I suspect it's related to an intensified need for reassurance and security from the spouse. In other instances, however, the increased sexual interest is almost certainly the direct result of the brain changes which are occurring.* Did Joe go through a stage of increased sexuality?"

"No . . . but he does need love."

"Nevertheless, you owe it to yourself and Joe, at this point, to begin considering a home. I'd better be going. Thank you for inviting me."

"Thank you for the medication . . . and the advice."

A week later Ilia called me. She was sobbing. "Joe lifted up a chair

---

* For example, there is a syndrome of hypersexuality accompanied by severe dementia, which is known to occur in primates following complete destruction of the temporal lobes on both sides of the head. This process involves total destruction of the amygdalae, the hippocampi, and the temporal neocortex and hence provides an extreme example of the pathology resulting from damage in the same brain areas as those affected by Alzheimer's disease. The pathological syndrome which results is marked by hypersexuality, dementia, and other changes, and is known as the Klüver-Bucy syndrome.[2] Other conditions associated with major brain pathology are also known to cause sexual changes including hypersexuality. Among these conditions are epilepsy and head trauma.[3]

to hit me. I had to put a table in front of the door to keep him from getting outside. He's never done anything like that. I don't know whether he would have actually struck me, but . . . ."

We agreed that Joe had to go into a home. Ilia found a skilled nursing facility which was sufficiently close to her and their children to permit frequent visits. Nine long weeks of waiting went by, and then an opening materialized and Joe was able to enter the home.

I visited Joe shortly after his arrival in the home. It was a bright, cheerful, fairly modern building. I was received by an alert, friendly registered nurse who complemented the surroundings. She directed me to Joe's room on the fourth floor. In the elevator one recognized a familiar, distinctive odor which is sometimes called "institutional." Ilia and I subsequently speculated that the aroma was a product of a combination of elements which accumulate in places where there are a large number of persons who are unable to care for themselves hygienically.

To the uninitiated, the floor onto which I emerged must have resembled a form of purgatory. Persons wandered about like shadows with vacant expressions which barely altered upon approach. The nursing station was directly opposite the elevators. Failing to find a nurse immediately, I set off down the corridor to search for Joe's room.

"Eee! Eee!" It was a high-pitched woman's voice. I turned around to see a tall, thin woman, about 85, with blond hair, wearing a loose-fitting print dress. She was being held by a Philippine nurse on one side and a black nursing attendant on the other.

"Catherine! Catherine!" the Philippine nurse cried. "I told you not to do that!" "Catherine's running away again," she informed another aide, a slightly built man dressed in a white shirt and trousers who came over to assist.

They pulled Catherine from the elevators and over to her room. I followed them down the hall. Catherine started to scream loudly.

"Catherine, now we've got to tie you down," the Philippine nurse explained evenly.

Catherine continued her screams as one of the aides moved to close the curtain around her bed.

"Oh, doctor," the Philippine nurse said calmly as she turned and saw me, "I'll be with you in a minute."

Feeling mildly intrusive, I turned down the corridor and resumed my search for Joe's room. I had no difficulty locating it. Joe was sitting in a chair staring blankly.

"Hello, Mr. S."

"Oh, hello."

"Do you know who I am?"

"You came to see me?"

"Yes, I'm Dr. Reisberg. Do you remember me?"

"No."

"I know you very well. Do you mind if I ask you some questions?"

"Well, all right."

"Okay. Then would you have a seat?"

"Okay." He sat down slowly.

"Mr. S., do you know what year it is?"

"Yes, it's . . . ." There was a long pause. Then Joe got up from the chair. He wandered over to the bathroom door. He opened and closed the door, then he started to wander out of the room. He seemed to have forgotten my presence.

"Mr. S., could you have a seat?"

"Okay," and he wandered slowly back to the chair.

"Could you sit down?"

"All right." He slowly sank back into the chair.

"Mr. S., I'd like you to count backwards from 20 by ones. Could you do that—20, 19, like that?"

"20, 19, 18, 17, 16, 15, 14, 13, 10, 20, 21, 22, 23, 24."

"What did I just ask you to do?"

"To count."

"From where?"

"From one."

"Mr. S., do you have any children?"

"I don't know."

"What are the names of your children?"

He got up from the chair and started to wander again.

"Mr. S., what is your wife's name?"

"Ilia."

"That's right, good. Where is she?"

"She is . . . with me."

"Uh, huh . . . and what kind of work did you used to do?"

"I . . . ." There was no further response. I put my hand on his shoulder. "Mr. S., could you sit down?"

He once again complied without difficulty.

"Mr. S., the year is 1979. Can you repeat that?"

"1979."

"Good."

"Do you remember who I am?"

"You are . . . yourself."

"That's right, I'm Dr. Reisberg. Do you know where you are?"

"I'm here."

"That's right. And where is this? Where is here?"

"Right here. That's all."

"Okay. Do you know what year this is?"

There was no answer. "Do you know the century? Around what year it is?"

Still no answer.

"It's 1979."

"Dr. Reisberg." I turned. It was the nurse with his chart.

"Thank you," I said, and began to look through it. Joe was receiving small doses of haloperidol, a powerful tranquilizer and sleeping medication in addition.

Haloperidol (Haldol) is a member of a class of drugs known as "antipsychotics." Other antipsychotic medications which are very frequently prescribed for elderly persons, particularly those in the dementia phase, are thioridazine (Mellaril), chlorpromazine (Thorazine), and trifluperazine (Stellazine). Another name for this class of pharmaceuticals, in addition to "antipsychotic," is "major tranquilizers."* In part because of the implications of the name "tranquilizer," these drugs are frequently prescribed by physicians to quiet elderly patients and to make them more manageable. Another way of describing the effects of these substances is as "chemical straightjackets."

Unfortunately, these compounds are actually very powerful and cause a whole constellation of side effects in addition to "tranquilization." For example, chlorpromazine and thioridazine, which are often prescribed indiscriminately to the elderly for "nervousness,"** frequently cause fainting and dizziness upon arising. Thioridazine is also a frequent cause of impotence and ejaculatory disturbances in elderly men.

When family members use terms such as "depression," and "anx-

---

* Other, more technical names for this class of compounds are "neuroleptics" and "ataractics." The terms "major tranquillizer," "neuroleptic," and "ataractic" usually refer to the same group of antipsychotic drugs.

** A recent study conducted among Medicaid patients in the state of California revealed that Mellaril was ranked first in terms of total drug expenditures among the institutionalized aged population.⁴ Mellaril alone accounted for 7.8 percent of drug expenditures among the institutionalized California Medicaid aged population.

iety'' to describe the behavior of elderly persons, they are frequently not using the terms in the medical sense, and hence ''antidepressants'' or ''antianxiety'' drugs are not necessarily indicated. At the same time, the family physicians and internal medicine specialists who frequently prescribe psychoactive drugs for the elderly are not expert themselves in diagnosing behavioral pathology and are often unaware of the precise indications for these drugs. Hence it appears they often ''try out'' these medications in response to the family members' complaints. This is most unfortunate, since unless these compounds are used properly and expertly, they undoubtedly cause more problems than they solve.

The major tranquilizer which Joe was receiving, haloperidol, frequently causes a syndrome of side effects which are known as ''Parkinsonian side effects'' because of their similarity to the effects of Parkinson's disease. These side effects include tremulousness, drooling, rigidity, and a shuffling gait. Persons suffering from these symptoms are commonly said to look like ''zombies,'' a resemblance accentuated by the wide staring eyes which are also a concomitant of the syndrome. These Parkinsonian side effects cause the confused or demented patient to look all the more confused and/or demented. Distinguishing the therapeutic effects of haloperidol from the side effects of the medication requires an expertise which few of the physicians prescribing the medication possess. And in any case, if the therapeutic goal was simply to sedate Joe and to minimize his anxiety, this could have been achieved with a *minor* tranquilizer, such as diazepam (Valium) or chlordiazepoxide (Librium), with considerably less hazard.

''He doesn't appear to be agitated. Does he need the Haldol?''

''You should see what he's like at other times, especially in the morning, and sometimes he starts waving his arms. He hit me on the wrist one time.''

''Why did he do that?''

''You know we have to shower him in the mornings. He can't do these things himself. He becomes very angry when we do these things. He starts swearing and cursing. You should be here.''

''Why do you think he's so angry in the mornings?''

''He doesn't like us to do these things for him. He wants to be left on his own.''

''I see. You know the Haldol may be contributing to the restlessness. It causes what we call an 'akathesia,' an inability to sit still. It can actually make people restless.''

"You can discuss that with Dr. Taylor."

"I will, but I'd like you to be aware of it. Also, those small shuffling steps he's taking may be from the Haldol, and he's showing some Parkinsonian rigidity to passive range of motion which is probably from the medication, although it may also be the result of deterioration in a certain portion of his brain."

"You can discuss all that with his doctor. There's a consultation sheet on the chart."

"How's his weight?"

"He's lost about seven pounds since he came here. We give him Sustacal twice a day. We have to keep telling him to eat, and sometimes we have to feed him."

"Does that work?"

"Sometimes . . . but he can become very angry and sometimes he'll push the food away or hit the person who's feeding him."

"It's a problem. Anyway, he doesn't seem to be starving. His skin is okay. There are no rashes. His cholesterol is normal, and there's no protein in his urine . . . so I suppose his nutritional status is more or less adequate. I notice he's getting multivitamins every day."

"Is there anything else I can do for you, doctor?"

"I agree with your concern that he eat adequately. He lost about 15 pounds during his hospitalization for the prostatic surgery. Unfortunately, it's very difficult to force someone to eat. Aside from his angry outbursts and his eating less, how has he reacted to being here?"

"He misses his wife. He asks for her all the time, day and night. He wanders from room to room asking for Ilia."

"Does she come often?"

"Almost every day."

"Does he do anything during the day? Does he participate in any activities? I noticed the physical therapy note, so apparently he's been evaluated for his ability to participate."

"No. He doesn't do anything in particular."

"Does he have any friends? Does he talk to anyone?"

"There is one man, Jake, who he sometimes says 'Hello' to."

"I don't suppose he can watch TV."

"No, he can't."

"Okay, thank you. I'll finish my consult and put the chart back in the nursing station when I'm through."

At that time there was very little that I could recommend apart from minimizing the amounts of tranquilizers being given to Joe and hence reducing some of the side effects resulting from these substances.

Joe remained in the nursing home. A year later, I received a call from Ilia.

"I'm thinking of taking Joe to a medium, Madame Rosa. Have you ever heard of her?"

"No."

"I spoke to her on the telephone. I explained Joe's situation to her. She said if his soul has not drifted too far away, she may be able to call him back. I don't know what to do. My daughter suggested I call you and ask your opinion, so . . . ."

"Joe would have no understanding of what was going on, and a few moments after the ritual was completed, he would have entirely forgotten that it ever had occurred."

"But if there's any chance, I would do anything."

"I know you would. There are people whom spiritualists and psychics can sometimes help, people whose illnesses have psychological components. Occasionally their results seem dramatic. For instance, they've ostensibly cured cancer victims. When medical scientists have studied the results, they have found that the victims believed themselves to have been cured and no longer complained of symptoms. However, the objective evidence of the pathology, for example the bloody urine or stools, remained. For illnesses which have a stronger psychological component and perhaps somewhat less of a physical basis than cancer, spiritualists' or psychics' cures can occasionally be even more impressive.

"Unfortunately, most psychological cures are dependent upon cognitive functioning. If the mind is functioning only minimally, the potential value of these cures is reduced concomitantly. How is Joe?"

"Well, he's on the medication and he's more subdued. Except in the morning—they tell me he's still belligerent in the morning and he swears at the nurses. I think it's because they're very insistent on what they want done. When they take him for a shower and bathe him, they want it done their way and at times which are convenient for them. That comes under the heading of restraint. Maybe he isn't ready for a shower or a shampoo just at the moment when they decide."

"Did he ever swear before?"

"Yes, but only in appropriate places. I mean, he wouldn't swear at somebody who was helping him. He wouldn't do that. He would swear if the story went badly or if he got wrong information from somewhere.

"In the nursing home, if he doesn't eat, because he forgets that he's eating and he'll stop, they'll either insist on his eating or they'll feed him. He doesn't want that. So he might say, 'Son of a bitch, take it away!' or something like that.''

''Has he had any illnesses or infections while he's been at the nursing home?''

''No.''

''How has his behavior changed over the part of the year that he's been in the nursing home?''

''When he first went into the home, he didn't want to stay. He made it very difficult for me to go home.''

''What would he say?''

''Well, he would say, 'Why are you leaving me here?' I . . . I . . . don't know if I can talk about it.'' Her voice began to crack.

''Say what you're feeling.''

''Well, he knew he was there, he knew he was in a home. I tried to tell him when he got well . . . when he got better . . . he could come home.

''One time he said to me, 'I don't do anything here. I don't go to the opera anymore, I don't go to the theater.' Which we did, at least two or three times a week before he went into the hospital.''

''Did he remember that?''

''Yes, he did. He said, 'I don't go to the opera, I don't go to the theater, there's nothing for me to do here and I don't know why I can't go home.' Then I would have to tell him that he was sick and that when he got better he could come home. Then, gradually, under the medication, it would seem that he would be more quiet when I came. Sometimes I would come and find him just staring and doing nothing. He gets that way more and more now.''

''You're right. That's probably from the medication.''

''He talks about things that make absolutely no sense.''

''Like what?''

''Well, the words don't come out right. Sometimes he says things that are not words. Like one time he said a very peculiar word and my son was there and he said, 'What does that mean, Dad?' Joe said, 'I'll spell it for you.' He spelled it the way he said it, but it wasn't a word.

''He's still writing stories in his head. He still talks about filing a story and getting it there on time. He also asks if his stories were all right and whether the editors were pleased. I go along with that and I tell him that I took the story to the editors, or took down the dictation, and he says, 'Have you got paper, have you got everything?' and I always assure him that I have.

"Of course, it's worse now and the words don't come out right, but once in a while he'll say things that make sense. This spring we were walking outdoors and everything was turning green, and I commented on how green everything looked and he said, 'Yes, I used to know how green was my valley.'

"He has a very good friend in the nursing home, his roommate who is just as confused as he is. They talk to each other about the most mixed-up, confused things. But they're very happy with this conversation."

"This is a roommate, you say?"

"Yes, he has been his roommate for several months."

"What's his name?"

"Jake, but Joe likes to call him Sam. But he answers to Sam. Jake answers to Sam, it doesn't bother him."

"That's very interesting. His name is Jake, but Joe likes to call him Sam?"

"That's right, because one of our very dearest friends was Sam, and he likes to call him Sam."

"That's amazing."

"And Jake doesn't mind . . . and Jake's in a wheelchair all the time and Joe is in a geriatric chair."

"What's a geriatric chair?"

"A geriatric chair is one with a tray in front of it. There are wheels and he has to move it with his legs. When I come or when the children come, we take him out of the chair and walk with him."

"How long does he have to stay in the chair?"

"All of the time, except if he is being showered or shaved. He can't get out of it. They're afraid he'll fall, so they keep him in the chair."

"Does he fall?"

"He fell twice. Once he hurt his toe and that caused him to fall and once he just sank down. He didn't hurt himself, he just lost control and sat on the floor. They became very upset because they're so afraid of him hurting himself, so they keep him in a chair. But I think his brain has just interrupted his motor control of his legs; it's as if he can no longer keep his legs going. That lasts about half a minute. He doesn't lose consciousness or anything, and then he'll start walking again. But they're scared; they're afraid that he'll really fall."

"He must be angry about being in the chair."

"Of course. In the morning, after they shower and bathe him, they put him in the chair. I think that's when he gets very angry and starts swearing.''

''Does he have any difficulty eating? Has he lost any more weight since going to the nursing home?''

''He's lost about another five pounds since your visit. But lately he's begun to have difficulty reaching for food. For example, if I bring him a banana, which he likes, he won't always take that banana from me. It's only been happening the past few weeks. It seems to me now that he doesn't always see it in the right place or he can't make his hand go to the right place. He also sits down very peculiarly lately. He has to put his hand out on the seat and I'm always afraid he'll miss it because he can't gauge the distance between his body and the chair.''

''Does he always recognize you?''

''Oh, yes. He always kisses me, always. And he talks to me, and the people who pass and say, 'How are you?' he'll say, 'I'm fine. How are you?' There are certain things that are on target, but then he'll go on and say something that makes no sense at all.

''The other day I said to him jokingly, 'Don't you love me anymore?'' He said, 'No, I don't.' I said, 'Why?' He said, 'Because you left me here.' That's the first time he ever said that. Of course, we still held hands and kissed goodbye. He's become very demonstrative. He never used to kiss me in public, but now he doesn't care who's around.''

''Can you tell me more about his relationship with Jake?''

''When Joe first went to the nursing home he met Jake, who was in another room. Whenever I came, I found Joe and Jake together, either in their chairs or Joe walking around near Jake and talking to him. For some reason, they found a lot to talk about. Jake is very quiet and very elegant-looking, with gray hair and a little gray moustache. He was in the manufacturing of coats. Jake is always busy with a customer. He's always fitting something, or selling something, or sending it somewhere. And for Joe, who was never anything but a cerebral person and who could never do anything with his hands, somehow Joe found it fascinating.

''Joe, in turn, was always writing a story and sending it off and meeting a deadline. I guess Jake listened to that, it was new for Jake.

''The two of them are just very happy together. They shake hands every time they see each other. Jake is always in a wheelchair. If I walk by with Joe, he puts his hand on Jake's shoulder and he gives him a pat.''

"How does Joe succeed in constantly writing stories?"

"In the beginning, when he first came, he had to have pencils and paper in his shirt pocket so that he would be ready for a story. It's something that he always had done, which he continued.

"Sometimes he'd be so insistent that I file the story that I'd have to leave the room with the paper, disappear for a minute or two, and come back and say, 'It's done.' "

"Did he write anything on the paper?"

"No, I don't think he could sign his name now."

"Does Joe have any relationships in the nursing home apart from Jake?"

"No."

"I take it that Jake has a similar problem."

"Yes, he does. His wife kept him at home with her when he was too confused to carry on a conversation. He also would pick the locks. He would take the screws out of the bolts that were holding the lock on the door so he could get out, he knew how to do that. Joe didn't know how to do that, but I think he would have."

"Do you think placing Joe in the nursing home has been a good choice for him?"

"Well, he gets more stimulation there than he would get at home. There are more people there and people talk to him, everybody likes him.

"I would rather have been able to have taken care of him at our home, had I been able to. I think he was very unhappy the first few months that he was there. I certainly am unhappy."

"Why?"

She began to cry. "I don't know. I . . . I just think, maybe, I could have taken care of him myself. Maybe I should have tried, but I couldn't afford 24-hour-a-day help.

"Anyway, he seems more content now then when he first went into the home. When he first arrived, he was impossible when I had to leave. He wanted to come with me and he couldn't understand why I was leaving him. But now, I explain to him that I have to catch a bus and I have to hurry, and he'll say, 'Go, you go, don't miss the bus,' and he sends me off, he kisses me goodbye . . . he seems more content." She began to cry again.

"Why do you feel so guilty?"

"Because he needs the love, he needs the care. If I put him to sleep with my arms around him, I think it would be good for him.

"I went once to the nursing home in the evening instead of during the day. I made the mistake of staying until they put him to bed. They put him to bed quite early. I kissed him goodnight, and it was terrible for him. He said, 'I don't want to sleep here unless you're going to stay. I want to go home with you.' It was so upsetting for him to have me there and yet for him to go to bed himself, because we've been married almost 50 years and we always slept together in a double bed. It's a way of life, that's all."

"How often do you visit now?"

"I go every day, except the two days that I work."

"Then you visit five days a week?"

"Yes."

"Well, it's clear to me that you've always done everything possible for Joe's welfare. I genuinely consider you a saint."

"Is there anything that you can recommend?"

"You've certainly done all you could. There are some medications which I could currently recommend. One is a vasodilator. Do you know whether he is receiving any medications of this type?"

"No."

"Well, there's no question that vasodilators improve the circulation of blood to the brain. There is some evidence, which is certainly preliminary, that senile persons who receive certain substances of this kind deteriorate less rapidly than those who do not receive the medication. This was the finding of a European study in which patients received the drug or a placebo for a 15-month period. The vasodilator-treated group showed less intellectual deterioration and less physiological deterioration.

"Could you discuss that with his attending physician?"

"I'll be pleased to."

"Is there anything else I can do?"

"There is also a dietary supplement which might be worthwhile, lecithin."

"I've heard of it. Is it really of any use?"

"We don't know yet for certain. We do know that there is a deficiency in a certain very important brain chemical called choline in persons with Joe's condition. It may be that replacing the chemical will improve the condition, or at least decrease the rate of deterioration. We won't know for certain whether replacing choline is of genuine benefit for years; in the interim, it might be worthwhile."

"What do I do?"

"Lecithin is the natural dietary source of choline. We know that it increases the blood concentration of choline, and it appears to increase the amounts of choline actually present in the brain."

"Okay, I'll buy some and give it to him when I visit. Do you think you can get the nurses to give him the lecithin regularly?"

"I'll see what I can do. I'll also try to get them to permit Joe to walk around more freely, without the geriatric chair."

"Oh, thank you. That would help."

"I'm pleased you called. Keep in touch."

"Thank you, doctor."

The authorities in the nursing home continued to require that Joe be confined to the geriatric chair. Hence Joe's anger and his vituperative outbursts continued. An additional real problem continued to be lack of communication between Joe and the staff members. The nursing aides and nursing assistants who were the principal persons associated with the day-to-day aspects of Joe's care had no specific training or instruction in the care of senile patients, although these patients comprise an absolute majority of persons in nursing homes. The problem in Joe's case was that they would do things to him, such as dress him and feed him, and not tell him what it was they were about to do. Joe's memory was sufficiently poor that he never really came to appreciate the routine procedures of the home. Hence Joe continued to interpret the aides' assistance with his daily activities as assaults upon his person. Accordingly, his anger continued unabated.

This vicious cycle, founded upon a fundamental lack of communication and empathy, might have gradually lessened over time if the same persons had continued to care for Joe. However, the vagaries of the rotating system were combined with a high rate of staff turnover, so that, for the most part, the nursing assistants responsible for Joe's care never really got to know him. One further demonstration of this lack of communication was the aides' continuous shouting at Joe. Although Joe's mind had deteriorated, his hearing remained intact. Hence it was not necessary to shout at Joe—only to talk to him and to explain what it was that one was planning to do to him.

Ilia continued to visit Joe frequently. He, in his own way, continued to anticipate and welcome her visits. The next six months were uneventful.

One-third of all persons who enter nursing homes die within the first year. Two-thirds are dead within three years.[5] Furthermore, it will be recalled that senility itself is associated with a decreased life expectancy. We have said that the senile are no more likely than other persons their age to suffer from arthritis, hearing loss, prostate problems, cancer, or the other medical conditions common to the elderly. Why, then, should their life expectancy be so low? The reason is that the senile are considerably more likely to develop conditions which afflict persons who are confined or unable to care for themselves.

Joe had survived a year and a half in the nursing home without developing any form of serious ailment in addition to his senility. Medically speaking, he was doing better than average. Undoubtedly, Ilia's frequent visits increased the staff's general vigilance and interest in Joe's health and well-being. Hence these visits were of tangible value to him physically as well as emotionally.

After 18 months in the home, Joe developed an ulceration on his ankle which did not heal. The ulceration was probably related to his confinement to the geriatric chair. Since Joe could not ambulate normally, the blood in his legs could not circulate properly. Ulcerations frequently develop under such conditions.

One month after the appearance of the ulcer, Joe's entire leg became swollen. The ulcer had worsened and was filled with fluid. Apparently, it had become infected and the infection was spreading. Joe was transferred to a hospital.

Joe remained in the hospital for 12 weeks. The wound was debrided, and he was treated with antibiotics. The staff, mercifully, agreed to minimal sedation. With antiseptic washes and proper care, the wound gradually healed. Ilia followed Joe to the hospital and maintained her vigilance. As always, her concern ensured him the proper attention and care.

Joe survived his medical crisis and returned to the nursing home. He continues to survive there. Unfortunately, his confinement and his anger also continue. Fortunately, so do Ilia's love and support. I have no doubt that Ilia's virtues are the primary factors responsible for Joe's survival. Confused though he is, I am also certain of Joe's awareness and appreciation of her love.

Notes

1. Reisberg, B., Ferris, S. H., and Gershon, S., Pharmacotherapy of senile dementia. In *Psychopathology in the Aged*, ed. by Jonathan O. Cole and James E. Barrett, Raven Press, New York, pp. 233–264, 1980.

2. Klüver, H., and Bucy, P. C., Preliminary analysis of the functions of the temporal lobes in monkeys. *Arch. Neurol. Psychiat.* 42: 979, 1939.

3. Small, I. F., and Small, J. G., Sexual behavior and mental illness. In *Comprehensive Textbook of Psychiatry/II,* ed. by A. M. Freedman, H. I. Kaplan, and B. J. Sadock, Williams & Wilkins, Baltimore, 1975, pp. 1500–1510.

4. Zawadski, R. T., Glazer, G. B., and Lurie, E., Psychotropic drug use among institutionalized and noninstitutionalized Medicaid aged in California. *J. Geront.* 33: 825–834, 1978.

5. Butler, R. N., *Why Survive? Being Old in America.* Harper & Row, New York, 1975, p. 269.

Chapter 7

Treating Alzheimer's Disease: Medical and Pharmacological Approaches

SURPRISINGLY, INTERVENTIONS which have been shown quite convincingly to be effective in reducing impairment in senile dementia already exist. Nonetheless, these treatments have not generated the excitement and enthusiasm which we would expect from the patients, their families, and their physicians. An understanding of this paradox requires some explanation.

Western medicine as an art and a discipline has traditionally focused on dramatic clinical improvement and rapid, seemingly sudden cures. This is not at all surprising, since these results are the ones most easily appreciated by patients and their relatives and they provide immediate satisfaction to the clinician. Unfortunately, these acute interventions are often merely palliative and temporary. At worst, they are simply "hocus-pocus," i.e., sufficiently dramatic as to seem magical but of little value other than to exaggerate the powers of physicians and of medical science in general.

Examples of these phenomena abound in each of the medical disciplines. For instance, in psychiatry physicians are frequently most impressively effective in relieving some of the side effects caused by the medications which they themselves give their patients. For example, patients sometimes develop muscle spasms in reaction to certain psy-

123

chotropic medications. By giving an antihistaminic agent intravenously, psychiatrists can dramatically relieve these spasms. The patients, their relatives, and all who witness the cure are understandably impressed. But all that has really been accomplished is the sudden relief of a symptom caused by the physician's medication in the first place. The underlying illness has not been affected at all. Furthermore, if the psychotropic medication is not discontinued, the spasms may return and recur repeatedly.

In neurology, another medical discipline which is frequently concerned with the diagnosis and therapy of senility, examples of the dramatic treatment of acute problems without actually affecting the underlying chronic ailment producing the problems are also readily available. One of the major therapeutic advances said to have occurred in this medical specialty over the past few decades has been in the treatment of Parkinson's disease. This condition is characterized by rigidity of movement, tremulousness, and, frequently, drooling. Cotzias discovered in the early fifties that giving a substance known as "L-dopa" dramatically relieved these symptoms. A seemingly miraculous cure had been found for a major illness in a medical specialty tragically lacking in effective interventions. Unfortunately, a quarter century later this dramatic discovery may have lost much of its significance. We now know that with time this dramatic "cure" becomes progressively less effective in "masking" the symptoms of this chronic disease, which lasts for the remainder of the patient's lifetime. Over the years, higher and higher doses of L-dopa or related substances are required to relieve the symptoms of the disease. The anti-Parkinsonian medication produces side effects which dilute the overall therapeutic benefit to the patient. With increasing dosages, the side effects may actually come to outweigh the therapeutic advantages to the patient. Unfortunately, the long-term course of the Parkinsonian disease does not seem to be affected by the dramatic symptomatic "cures" which are available.[1]

In certain ways the modern medical approach to healing is analogous to more traditional "spiritual" techniques. An interesting investigation was conducted of fundamentalist Christian spiritual "cures" among American believers suffering from cancer. These "cures" are effected by so-called "laying on of hands" on persons who are "true believers" in the potential efficacy of the procedure. The cancer sufferers who were included in the study believed that they had been cured as a result of the ritual. Indeed, they were found to have achieved symptomatic relief. They no longer experienced the physical or psychological discomfort which had developed with the spread of the malignancy. Hence, from the believers' viewpoint they were "cured." However, the physical manifestations of the cancer continued. The signs of bleeding in the urine or in the stools continued as before. The inexorable progression of the cancer was not affected by the spiritual "cures."[2]

In recent years the medical and scientific establishments have become increasingly aware of the need for Western medicine to concern itself more with the prevention and long-term amelioration of chronic disease. However, our hospital-centered medical system remains primarily concerned with dampening the flames of acute "flare-ups" of illness. The long-term treatment and prevention of chronic disease continue to receive much less attention.

Senility is, of course, a chronic illness. A truly important and effective agent for this condition is one which can favorably alter its course and progression over the years. A "hocus-pocus" palliative which reverses symptoms for only a short while and has no real effect on the long-term course of the disorder will undoubtedly attract more attention and excitement but will be of less real significance. Fortunately, it appears that substances which are effective in favorably altering the gradual decline which occurs in senile dementia may have already been developed. These potentially significant compounds have received less than adequate attention from laymen, their families, and even physicians, for the reasons described above.

A wide variety of drugs have been investigated in the treatment of senility. Among the most important, the most widely known, and the most promising substances which have been investigated are the following:

I. Cerebral vasodilators and cerebral metabolic enhancers
II. Procaine solution
III. Psychostimulants
IV. Nootropics
V. Neuropeptides
VI. Neurotransmitter precursors or agonists

The cerebral vasodilators and the cerebral metabolic enhancers are the most important and the most widely used substances in the treatment of brain failure. The reasoning behind the use of these substances has changed as our conceptions of the origins of senile dementia have shifted. When the vasodilator treatments were first introduced, senility was thought to be the result of the progressive narrowing of the blood vessels in the brain by the build-up of arteriosclerotic deposits. The vasodilators were thought to assist in the treatment of this progressive cerebral arteriosclerosis by expanding the narrowed blood vessels.

As we have seen, our conceptions regarding the origins of senile dementia have changed dramatically. We now believe that a degenerative condition, Alzheimer's disease, is the cause of a majority of cases of senile dementia, and that a vascular condition, multi-infarct dementia, is responsible for a majority of the remaining instances of senility. Multi-infarct dementia, unlike Alzheimer's disease, is associated with arteriosclerosis in the blood vessels throughout the body.

What do these new conceptions of the origins of senile dementia mean in terms of the rationale and utility of the vasodilator therapies? Recent experiments reveal some surprising implications.

Carbon dioxide is a powerful natural dilator of the cerebral blood vessels. Our bodies appear to have developed this natural adaptive response because a build-up in carbon dioxide concentration generally indicates that our tissues are not getting sufficient oxygen. The brain is one of the most sensitive organs in our body to lack of oxygen. The brain can develop permanent damage in a relatively short time from insufficient oxygen. Therefore, the body has developed a variety of mechanisms for shunting blood to the brain in times of need. One of these mechanisms is the vasodilatory response of the cerebral vessels to an increased carbon dioxide concentration.

Experiments indicate that patients with Alzheimer's disease can respond at least as well as expected to a vasodilatory stimulus such as carbon dioxide (see figure 7-1). The vessels expand and there is an increase in blood flow. In fact, patients with Alzheimer's disease appear to show a slightly greater response to a vasodilatory stimulus than do unimpaired, normal persons of the same age. Multi-infarct dementia patients have cerebral blood vessels which are frequently sclerosed. The arteriosclerotic deposits create rigid blood vessels which are incapable of expanding. Indeed, many of the vessels become like lead pipes—rigid and virtually immobile. Experiments confirm that vasodilatory substances have very different effects in multi-infarct dementia patients with these rigid, sclerosed vessels. Multi-infarct dementia patients do not show an increase in cerebral blood flow in response to cerebral vasodilators. In fact, these patients actually show a slight decrease in blood flow. Apparently, the only direction in which

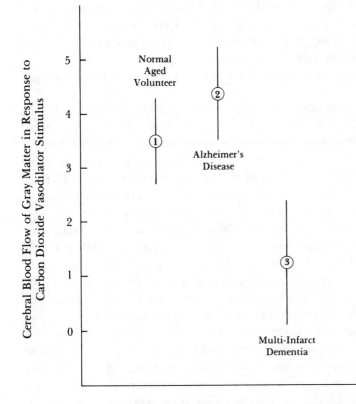

Carbon Dioxide Responsiveness of Cerebral Blood
Flow of Gray Matter in (1) Normal Aged Volunteers,
(2) Alzheimer's Disease Patients, and (3) Multi-
infarct Dementia Patients

Figure 7.1 Cerebral Blood Flow Responsiveness in Aging and Dementia
Source: Modified from Yamaguchi et al., "Noninvasive cerebral blood flow measurements in dementia." Arch. Neurol. *1980, 37: 410–418.*

these rigid, sclerotic blood vessels are capable of moving is inward, and this is indeed the paradoxical response which they show in response to a dilatory stimulus.[3]

These findings indicate that vasodilator agents may be therapeutic in cases of dementia due to Alzheimer's disease, but may be of no benefit and possibly cause a slight worsening in patients with dementia due to multi-infarct dementia. Unfortunately, no drug studies have been conducted which comparatively analyzed the effects of the cerebral vasodilator substances in these two very different dementia types. Negative effects of cerebral vasodilators in patients with multi-infarct dementia may tend to obscure positive effects in the Alzheimer's patients. If this diluting effect is indeed occurring, then the reports of treatment response with the vasodilator therapies may prove to be of even greater significance when these agents are used in appropriate patient subgroups.

The vasodilator which is the most widely used and which has been studied most intensively in the treatment of senility is known technically as "dihydroergotoxine." It is a substance derived from a fungus which grows on rye bread and other cereal grains. A study recently conducted among Medicaid recipients in the state of California revealed that this compound ranked second in terms of total drug expenditures among that state's institutionalized population.[4]

More than 100 clinical studies of the efficacy of dihydroergotoxine in the treatment of diverse groups of elderly patients with thinking disturbances have been conducted (for reviews see reference notes 5, 6, and 7). These studies indicate positive effects of the substance in the treatment of many of the clinical symptoms frequently observed among these patients. Specifically, the symptoms of lack of alertness, poor orientation, confusion, weak recent memory, depressed mood, anxiety, lack of motivation, agitation, dizziness, and poor ability to move around have all shown improvement. Furthermore, the better designed a study is, in scientific terms, the more likely it is to demonstrate improvement. The magnitude of the improvement in these various symptoms is small; that is to say, the changes produced are not dramatic. The great majority of studies of dihydroergotoxine's clinical efficacy have lasted no longer than three months. Interestingly, analysis seems to reveal continuing improvement throughout that three-month period.

We have discussed the importance of long-term effects in the treatment of chronic illnesses such as senile dementia. The effects of a treatment on the course of a chronic illness over several months or several years may be more important than dramatic effects observed the day after a treatment is begun. It is interesting and perhaps significant that dihydroergotoxine seems to gradually show greater and greater efficacy over the course of the first three months of treatment. What are its effects over treatment periods extending for several months or even longer?

Unfortunately, it appears that no studies extending for longer than a six-month period have been done in this country. However, there is an intriguing and very encouraging European study which lasted for 15

T A B L E 7-1. Long-Term Hydergine Treatment Study

NURSING HOME RESIDENTS 4.5 MG HYDERGINE/DAY	PLACEBO	EXPERIMENTALS
6 mos	No significant difference in general intelligence	No significant difference in general intelligence
	↑ in cerebral circ time	↓ in cerebral circ time
15 mos	↓ in general intelligence	5–7% ↑ in general intelligence
	↑↑ in cerebral circ time	↓ in cerebral circ time
	↑ in power range for frequencies analyzed on EEG	↓ in power range for frequencies analyzed on EEG

Source: Kugler, J., Oswald, W. D., Herzfeld, U., Seus, R., and Ringel, J., Long-term treatment of the symptoms of senile cerebral insufficiency: A prospective study of Hydergine, *Dtsch. Med. Wschr,* 103:456–462, 1978.

months[8] (see Table 7-1). This study, which was conducted among nursing home residents, employed dosages of 4.5 milligrams of dihydroergotoxine daily, a slightly larger amount than the three milligrams daily which are customarily recommended. After six months of treatment there were no evident differences in a test of general intelligence from the results obtained at the beginning of the study, either for patients who received dihydroergotoxine treatment or for those treated with placebo. This is not really surprising, since, as we have seen, senile dementia has a very gradual downhill course. In contrast, after 15 months of treatment the placebo-treated patients showed a decline in general intelligence, just as we would expect. However, the group of nursing home residents receiving the dihydroergotoxine treatment actually showed a slight *increase* in performance in the intelligence test over the 15-month period!

Certain objective tests of physiological changes further support the apparent long-term value of dihydroergotoxine treatment. Cerebral blood flow declined at six months in the nursing home residents who received placebo. In patients with Alzheimer's disease, the decline in blood flow to the brain appears to occur secondarily, as a result of the gradual destruction of the neurons. The remaining functional brain cells are fewer in number and therefore require less oxygen and nourishment. Blood flow decreases because of this reduced need.

Expectedly, after 15 months, blood flow to the brain declined even further among the patients who received placebo. However, the dihydroergotoxine-treated patients showed an improvement in brain circulation as a result of this vasodilator treatment. The improvement in the brain's blood flow was evident after six months of treatment and was still present after 15 months of treatment.

Another source of objective evidence for the long-term value of treatment with the ergot derivative comes from studies of the electrical activity of the brain. Any process which causes marked brain changes, particularly to the outer layers, or cortex, of the brain, will alter its electrical activity. Scientists can record the brain's electrical activity using electroencephalograms or similar devices. The characteristics of the electrical activity can then be studied in great detail.

Alzheimer's disease produces certain kinds of changes in the brain's electrical activity, and they become more pronounced over the years. The progression of electrical changes in Alzheimer's disease was observed in the placebo-treated nursing home residents. However, the residents who received dihydroergotoxine did not have more pronounced changes in electrical activity after 15 months. Indeed, the changes seen in the treated patients were in the opposite direction from those observed in the untreated group.

Hence there is convincing preliminary evidence that the vasodilator dihydroergotoxine is of long-term value in the treatment of senile dementia. Future studies which distinguish between the Alzheimer's dementia and the multi-infarct dementia subgroups may demonstrate even greater utility for this agent in the treatment of Alzheimer's disease. Also, the proper dosage of dihydroergotoxine, the dosage which will produce the maximum therapeutic benefit, needs to be determined. These "dose response" studies are yet to be conducted. Finally, studies extending for two years and longer need to be conducted to determine the genuine long-term value of dihydroergotoxine treatment.

Other chemical substances which are known to improve the blood circulation to the brain have also shown value in the treatment of brain failure. An example is papaverine, which is marketed as Pavabid©. Papaverine is found in opium. Despite its origin it does not have any narcotic properties. It does cause relaxation of involuntary muscles and has been shown to increase blood flow to the brain. At least four scientifically sound studies have found papaverine to be of value in the treatment of mixed groups of senile patients.[9,10,11,12]

As we have seen, dihydroergotoxine appears to have increased clinical efficacy with increased duration of treatment; there is some evidence that the same holds true for papaverine treatment. In one study, investigators found that definite improvement tended to occur after a year and a half to two years of treatment.[11] These positive changes with papaverine treatment were reflected in measures of the brain's electrical activity. After two years of treatment with papaverine, half of the patients treated had changes in the EEG (electroencephalogram) in the direction of normality. The other 50 percent of the patients who received papaverine showed no marked changes on the EEG over the two-year period. In contrast, two-thirds of the EEGs of placebo-treated patients showed changes indicating deterioration.

Clinical investigations which have compared treatment with papaverine with treatment with dihydroergotoxine have found the latter to be superior.[13,14] However, these comparisons only extended over a few months and were in diverse senile populations.

Other marketed, currently available vasodilator drugs have also been shown to be of value in the treatment of diverse groups of senile dementia patients. These include cyclandelate (Cyclospasmol©, Ives Laboratories) and isoxsuprine (Vasodilan©). However, the current evidence for the utility of these substances is much less convincing than that currently available for dihydroergotoxine, or even papaverine.

Although we have referred to the agents mentioned thus far—dihydroergotoxine, papaverine, cyclandelate, and isoxsuprine—by the customary generic term "vasodilator," the primary therapeutic action of these agents may not be vasodilation. For example, they may improve the metabolism and functioning of the brain cells and, consequently, lead to increased cerebral blood flow secondarily. Indeed, some substances customarily classified as vasodilators are currently believed to function primarily as metabolic enhancers. An example is naftidrofuryl (Praxilene©), a drug which is currently marketed in Europe and which is under investigation in the United States. Naftidrofuryl has been shown to increase the energy stored by the brain. It may accomplish this by activating an enzyme which is important in the cellular production of energy from substances such as glucose. Naftidrofuryl increases cerebral blood flow secondarily, by first increasing the amount of energy in the brain. It too has shown promise in the treatment of senile dementia.[15,16,17,18,19,20]

Another form of treatment, which is based on the hypothesis that improved cerebral supply of oxygen can improve the symptoms of senile dementia, is hyperbaric oxygen treatment. This consists of sessions in which patients are placed in a chamber where they are exposed to oxygen under increased pressure. Although initial positive results were reported for this procedure,[21,22,23,24,25,26] careful scientific investigation has not shown it to be of value.[27,28]

Nevertheless, hyperbaric oxygen treatment has continued in many places and receives occasional attention from the media.[29,30] It has been estimated that there are currently approximately 100 hyperbaric oxygen (HBO) chambers in the United States. Typically, treatment consists of 10 to 20, or more sessions in the chamber. Each session lasts approximately one to two hours. The drama and the attention associated with the procedure are such that it would be expected to have a considerable nonspecific, or "placebo," effect. This effect probably accounts for the uncontrolled reports of the procedure's efficacy.

Gerovital-H3 (G-H3), or "Rumanian procaine," is another treatment which continues to enjoy popularity, despite a paucity of scientific data to justify the broad claims made by the solution's proponents. G-H3 was developed by Dr. Ana Aslan, a Rumanian physician, and it has been utilized in that country for more than a quarter century. Dr. Aslan has claimed a very wide range of therapeutic effects for the solution, effects which may be said to fall within the category of "rejuvenation."[31,32,33]

The solution consists of 2 percent procaine hydrochloride. Procaine (better known as Novocaine) is said to be the active ingredient. Procaine has many pharmacological properties. It is well known for its anesthetic properties and is a commonly used local anesthetic. The chemical property which is probably most closely related to its use in aging is its ability to decrease, or "inhibit," the action of an enzyme known as monoamine oxidase or MAO. This enzyme breaks down certain kinds of neurotransmitter substances.

The neurotransmitters, as we have said earlier, are the chemical messengers by which nerve cells communicate with one another. These chemical messengers must be rapidly broken down so that new messages can be transmitted. One of the major enzymes responsible for that breakdown is MAO.

Psychiatrists believe that certain kinds of severe depression are caused by a lack or depletion of neurotransmitter chemicals in certain parts of the brain. They believe that these depressions can be treated by increasing the quantities of the depleted neurotransmitters. One way this can be accomplished is by preventing the neurotransmitter breakdown by agents such as MAO. Hence an "MAO inhibitor" is a substance which can prevent the breakdown of certain kinds of neurotransmitters and which may thereby serve as an antidepressant. Indeed, many drugs which are used by psychiatrists for the treatment of depression are MAO inhibitors.

This MAO-inhibitory property, with its resulting antidepressant effect, appears to explain the action of G-H3. MAO activity is known to increase with aging. This increased activity may help to explain the increased incidence of severe depressions as people age. Procaine solution appears to be capable of blocking part of the increase in MAO activity and consequently useful in treating certain kinds of age-related depressions. Indeed, recent chemical trials have indicated that G-H3 may be of value in the treatment of depression among the aged.[34,35,36]

G-H3 may have favorable effects on mood and may ultimately prove of value in treating the minority of aged persons whose memory problems are the result of a primary mood disturbance. Unfortunately, however, there exists little or no good evidence of its benefit for the memory and thinking disturbances which plague persons with senile dementia.

The psychostimulants are compounds which are known popularly as "uppers." Among the psychostimulants are the amphetamines, which include such well-known substances as Benzedrine© (Smith, Kline, and French) (amphetamine sulfate) and Dexedrine© (Smith, Kline and French) (dextroamphetamine sulfate). These compounds are thought to possess properties which in theory might be supposed to have beneficial effects in senile persons. For example, they are thought to "elevate mood" and "enhance attention." Indeed, two of the psychostimulant compounds are listed in the *Physician's Desk Reference* (PDR), the popular and authoritative clinician's guide to drug prescribing, as being effective or as "possibly effective" in the treatment of aged patients with symptoms of senility.[37]

Unfortunately, these substances have not fulfilled their promise in the alleviation of disturbances associated with senility. For example, the United States Food and Drug Administration (FDA) recently reviewed the evidence for the clinical efficacy of the two compounds listed in the PDR, methylphenidate (Ritalin ©, Ciba) and pentylenetetrazol (Metrazol ©, Knoll and others). "In relation to the treatment of senility, the consensus was 'lacking substantial evidence of effectiveness.' "[38] Nevertheless, data indicate that approximately one of every seven prescriptions written by U.S. private practitioners for methylphenidate is for the treatment of the symptoms of senility. Other psychostimulant compounds continue to enjoy some popularity in this area as well. Hence a brief review as to why these seemingly promising substances do not appear to be effective may be useful.

A surprising finding is that the "psychostimulant" compounds do not necessarily have the effects on the brain and on behavior which we would expect. For example, when an ordinary, "therapeutic" dosage of the popular psychostimulant dextroamphetamine was given to adult volunteers in one study, there were some very surprising results. More than half of the volunteers were found to be *drowsy* an hour after the "stimulant." Measures of the electrical activity of the brain confirmed a loss in alertness in these volunteers. After two hours all of the volunteers did become more alert than they had been when they first took the "upper." However, the inescapable conclusion is that "amphetamine is not a simple stimulant of the . . . nervous system, but can also act as a depressant."[39]

The important question for our purposes is, what are the effects of the psychostimulants methylphenidate and pentylenetetrazol, which are sometimes said to have value in treating senile dementia?

My associates conducted a very careful study of this question with the frequently used stimulant methylphenidate. They found no genuine differences in thinking or performance between patients who received placebo and those who received methylphenidate. Furthermore, a broad range of dosage strengths of the "stimulants" appeared to be equally ineffective.[40]

For pentylenetetrazol, the current evidence is almost equally unencouraging. A majority of studies of this substance in persons with intellectual impairment and confusion have not indicated efficacy.[41]

A very promising substance which may prove to be a valuable treatment of brain failure is a new drug known as piracetam (Nootropil ©, UCB). Piracetam appears to be a unique compound, unrelated to any of the thousands of pharmaceutical substances which are currently available.[42]

In early investigations with piracetam, the drug appeared to improve the learning ability of animal subjects. It also appeared to protect the animals against the forgetting which ordinarily occurs under conditions of low oxygen. Among the substance's most interesting effects were the changes it induced in the brain's electrical activity. It increased the electrical activity in the portion of the brain which carries impulses between the cerebral hemispheres. Hence it was postulated that piracetam decreased the time which it would ordinarily take for information to go from one side of the head to the other!

There were other unusual properties which pointed to the apparent uniqueness of this new compound. For instance, we know that virtually all pharmaceuticals, those chemical substances which have therapeutically useful actions on the body's functioning, have side effects, other effects of the drug on bodily functioning which occur apart from the therapeutic action. A well-known example is aspirin, which may cause stomach bleeding apart from its ability to relieve a headache. Piracetam has definite effects on the functioning of the brain; however, it has never been found to have side effects, either in people or in animals. Nor does the drug have pain-reducing, sleep-producing, or calming effects, which are common properties of compounds which affect the mind. Conversely, it does not produce an increase in heart rate, respiration, or blood pressure. Even cerebral blood flow has not been found to change with piracetam treatment. One thing piracetam may do in common with some of the other substances which we mentioned earlier, however, is to increase the quantity of energy stored by the brain.

In an early study, piracetam was given to English college students who were studying for an exam. One group of students received a placebo, and another group took the actual drug. The group of students who took the piracetam did considerably better on the exam![43]

Subsequent studies with unimpaired older adults[44] and with persons with mild to moderate age-related thinking disturbances[45] have supported the ability of piracetam to improve thinking and behavior in these groups of people. Piracetam has not been shown to be of benefit in persons with severe "dementia stage" illness.[45,46,47]

Hence piracetam would appear to be of possible value in persons in the early and middle stages, that is, the "forgetfulness" and "confused" stages, of senile dementia. It is currently marketed and in use in many areas of the world. In the United States it is currently available for investigational purposes. Investigations should give us more conclusive information as to whether the drug is truly effective in treating senility. Of course, for the substance to truly be of value, long-term positive effects must be demonstrated, and investigations of long-term effects are currently years away. It is possible that piracetam will be the forerunner of a new class of drugs whose effects are primarily on thinking. In fact, a name for this group of substances, "nootropics" ("NOOΣ," meaning "mind," and "TPOΠEIN," meaning "toward"), has already been proposed. Hopefully, scientists will be able to develop even more powerful nootropics which may ultimately improve thinking ability in most aged persons and perhaps even in the young.

Another group of substances which has attracted considerable attention and caused a good deal of excitement in the past few years, and which may prove to be of value in treating senility and thinking disturbances in general, is the "neuropeptides." These are simple compounds composed of amino acids, the building blocks from which proteins are formed. Short chains of amino acids are known as "peptides," and many of these peptides have been found to profoundly affect the nervous system, hence the term "neuropeptides." Certain kinds of neuropeptides have been found to act as hormones and transmitters in the nervous system and elsewhere, serving to communicate instructions and messages between body cells, tissues, and organs. One group of these neuropeptides appears to control the perception of pain sensation by the brain. New roles of these substances in mediating bodily function are being discovered at such a rate that the prestigious *New England Journal of Medicine* stated in a recent editorial that "the neuropeptides, in particular, represent what might be described in the New York Stock Exchange as a growth area."[48]

The original basis for the scientific interest in the neuropeptides in the reversal of memory impairment came from certain intriguing experiments with animals. It was discovered that removal of the pituitary gland from certain animals decreased their learning ability[49] (see Figure 7-2). The pituitary is one of the most important glands in the body. As the so-called "master gland," it is the source of hormones which influence other glands such as the adrenals, the thyroid, and the

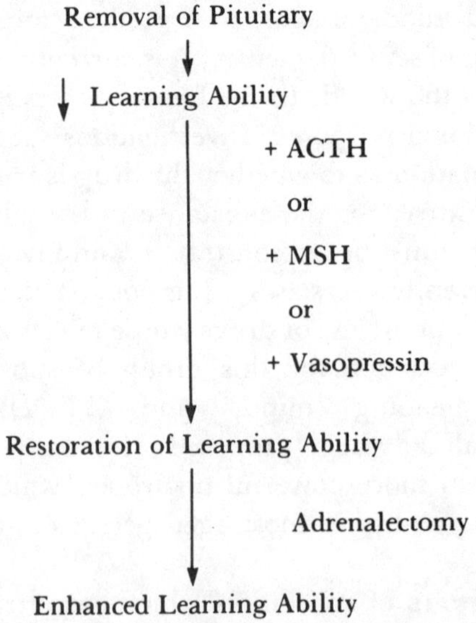

Removal of Pituitary
↓
↓ Learning Ability

+ ACTH

or

+ MSH

or

+ Vasopressin

Restoration of Learning Ability

Adrenalectomy

Enhanced Learning Ability

Figure 7.2   Hormonal Effects on Avoidance Learning in Animals

sex glands, as well as being the source of other hormones which influence bodily functions directly. Surprisingly, it was found that certain *individual* hormones were capable of reversing the loss of learning ability produced by the removal of the entire pituitary gland. These individual hormones were adrenocorticotropic hormone (ACTH), melanocyte-stimulating hormone (MSH), and vasopressin.[50,51]

ACTH is the pituitary hormone which stimulates the adrenal glands. Why should a substance such as this have effects on learning? Do the learning effects of ACTH relate to its stimulation of the adrenals?

Scientists had a simple means with which to answer these questions. They removed the adrenal glands and observed the resulting effects on learning in the animals. If the adrenal effects of ACTH had any relationship to its memory effects, then removal of the adrenal glands should counteract the ability of ACTH to improve learning ability. This did not occur. In fact, removing the adrenal glands actually increased the powers of ACTH to restore learning ability (presumably because of the increase in circulating ACTH which occurs after removal of the adrenal glands).[52] Hence the effects of ACTH on learning ability appeared to be independent of its effects on the adrenal glands. The hormone appeared to act directly on the brain in such a manner as to improve learning ability.

Another very interesting observation was that melanocyte-stimulating hormone (MSH) appeared to be as effective as ACTH in improving learning ability in the animals after removal of the pituitary gland. MSH ordinarily influences the pigment cells, or melanocytes, in our bodies. It is this hormone which provides the signal for our skins to turn darker when we lie in the sun.

What does this have to do with learning and memory?

Subsequent work demonstrated that a particular fragment of the ACTH molecular structure was able to account for all of the compound's memory effects. This fragment consisted of only seven amino acids. Furthermore, exactly the same seven-amino-acid sequence is found in the MSH molecule. Eventually, it was demonstrated that it was possible to reduce the fragment to as little as a four-amino-acid sequence and still maintain its learning properties.[53,54]

Human experiments on the improvement of learning ability with these fragments of the ACTH (or, if one prefers, MSH) molecule have not yielded encouraging results suggesting clinical utility in the near future.[55,56,57] However, vasopressin, the other peptide substance which was found to reverse the learning disabilities produced by removal of the pituitary, appears to be quite promising, and may prove to be the first of these neuropeptide substances which will be used to improve thinking capacity.

Apart from its ability to reverse learning deficits after pituitary surgery, other observations in animals support the ability of vasopressin to affect memory. There is a strain of rats born with a congenital genetic defect which makes the animals incapable of producing vasopressin. These animals are unable to retain the memories of new responses in which they have been trained.[58] If we inject the missing vasopressin into these animals, their learning ability improves.[59] Even more astounding is the ability of scientists to get rats to "remember" responses they have previously forgotten by injecting vasopressin.[60]

The preliminary human experiments conducted with vasopressin are also a source of optimism. When a vasopressin nasal spray was given to people with memory disturbances, their memories appeared to return more quickly.[61] Another more carefully controlled study found that adult men receiving vasopressin showed improved attention, concentration, and recall.[62] Further studies will tell us whether or not vasopressin will indeed prove to be of value in senility and other memory and thinking disorders.

Another group of neuropeptides, known as the "enkephalins," may also someday prove to be useful in improving thinking and memory. The enkephalins are recently discovered, natural substances which are normally present in the brain. They seem to play an important role in our experiencing painful sensations. Animal experiments also indicate that these substances may affect memory in much the same way as vasopressin.[63]

Many scientists believe that the neuropeptides are the actual substances which are used to communicate certain kinds of messages between many of the brain's neurons. As such, neuropeptides might be the chemicals which stimulate certain kinds of neurons to "remember." If these theories are correct, then the neuropeptides—vasopressin, the enkephalins, and perhaps others—may provide an important key to the unlocking of lost memories and the improvement of learning and thought.

Considering what has been discussed regarding the possible role of certain peptide substances as special "neurotransmitters" and regarding the possible cognitive consequences of "neurotransmission," it is not surprising that the major traditional neurotransmitter systems have been implicated in thinking processes in general and in senility in particular. Of these, the cholinergic system has recently been singled out as perhaps being a primary locus of Alzheimer's-disease-related memory impairment.

In Chapter 3 we reviewed some of the evidence implicating the cholinergic neurotransmitter system in Alzheimer's disease. It will be recalled that CAT, an enzyme which is concerned with the manufacture of acetylcholine in the body, was found to be decreased in activity in persons with Alzheimer's disease but not in persons with senile dementia of other origins. Further evidence of a relationship was the finding that the decrease in CAT activity appeared to correspond to the severity of the Alzheimer's dementia. We also described how substances which block acetylcholine, known as "anticholinergics," can produce memory impairments very similar to those observed in senile dementia.

Naturally, agents which increase the quantity of acetylcholine in the brain have been investigated in the treatment of senility in general and of Alzheimer's disease in particular. One method of increasing the quantity of acetylcholine in the body is with the direct administration of choline salts. These substances can be readily ingested orally and have been investigated at several centers. The results of treatment with choline salts currently appear disappointing.[64] My associates and I are conducting a major investigation of these agents with the support of the National Institute of Mental Health, which may provide a final answer regarding the utility of choline salt treatment in dementia patients.[65]

The natural dietary substance lecithin appears to be a better source of choline for the body organs, particularly for the brain, than the choline salts themselves.[66] Lecithin is a complex, fatty substance which is present in many foods, such as egg yolks, meat, and fish. The lecithin which is sold in health food stores and which has been tested for therapeutic benefit is derived from soy beans. Lecithin contains a substance called "phosphatidyl choline" which is present in the membranes of our cells, and which is thought to be the natural dietary source of choline.

Hence there is reason to believe that the ingestion of foods which contain lecithin will result in increased quantities of choline in the brain and that, in persons with Alzheimer's disease who have a deficiency of choline, the lecithin may help to improve thinking processes. One study based upon this hypothesis has been published, and the results suggested improvement in three of the seven Alzheimer's disease patients who received lecithin.[67] Other studies with larger numbers of patients must be conducted. However, the possibility of using natural dietary substances in the treatment of Alzheimer's disease has already aroused considerable excitement.

Another promising approach has been to employ other chemical substances which can stimulate the neuronal response to acetylcholine in the treatment of Alzheimer's patients. One such substance is physostigmine, a chemical which inhibits the enzyme which destroys acetylcholine released at the synapse. By this action, physostigmine produces an effective increase in the acetylcholine neurotransmitter substance. Experiments currently indicate that physostigmine *can* improve thinking ability in persons with Alzheimer's disease and other conditions. However, the relationship seems to be very delicate, and either too much or too little physostigmine is nontherapeutic.[68]

Logically, physostigmine and lecithin have been tried in combination. The preliminary results appeared to be beneficial.[69]

Hence we are probably justified in optimistically anticipating the time when Alzheimer's disease will be treated primarily by ingesting the proper foods, probably in combination with appropriate drugs. But where does this bring us to presently? What substances can reasonably be recommended now for the treatment of Alzheimer's disease?

The cerebral vasodilators and metabolic enhancers in general have been demonstrated, on the basis of the information currently available, to be of use in arresting or decreasing the decline ordinarily seen in Alzheimer's disease.

These substances will not ease the illness. However, they probably can prevent it from getting worse as rapidly as it otherwise would. In the near future we may be in a position to recommend the addition of other agents, such as lecithin. However, for the present, the recommendation of the cerebral vasodilators and metabolic enhancers probably represents the limits of what can be supported by scientific evidence.

Notes

1. Yahr, M. D., Long-term levodopa in Parkinson's disease (letter). *Lancet* 1(8013): 706-7, Mar. 26, 1977.
2. Pattison, E. M., Lapins, N. A., and Doerr, H. A., Faith healing: A

study of personality and functioning. *J. Nerv. Ment. Dis.* Vol. 157, No. 6, 397–409, December 1973.

3. Yamaguchi, F., Meyer, J. S., Yamamoto, M., Sakai, F., and Shaw, T., Noninvasive cerebral blood flow measurements in dementia, *Arch. Neurol.* 37: 410–418, 1980.

4. Zawadski, R. T., Glazer, G. B., and Lurie, E., Psychotropic drug use among institutionalized and noninstitutionalized Medicaid aged in California. *J. Geront.* 33: 824–834, 1978.

5. Hughes, J. R., Williams, J. G., and Currie, R. D., An ergot alkaloid preparation (hydergine) in the treatment of dementia: Critical review of the clinical literature. *J. Amer. Geriatrics Soc.* 24: 490–497, 1976.

6. Yesavage, J. A., Tinklenberg, J. R., Hollister, L. E., and Berger, P. A., Vasodilators in senile dementias. *Arch. Gen. Psychiat.* 36: 220–223, 1979.

7. Reisberg, B., Ferris, S. H., and Gershon, S., Pharmacotherapy of senile dementia, in J. O. Cole and J. E. Barrett (eds.), *Psychopathology in the Aged,* pp. 233–264, Raven Press, New York, 1980.

8. Kugler, J., Oswald, W. D., Herzfeld, U., Seus, R., and Ringel, J., Long term treatment of the symptoms of senile cerebral insufficiency: A prospective study of hydergine. *Dtsch. Med. Wschr.* 103: 456–462, 1978.

9. Stern, F. H., Management of chronic brain syndrome secondary to cerebral arteriosclerosis with special reference to papaverine hydrochloride. *J. Amer. Geriatrics Soc.* 18: 507–512, 1970.

10. Ritter, R. H., Nail, H. R., Tatum, P., and Blazi, M., The effect of papaverine on patients with cerebral arteriosclerosis. *Clin. Med.* 78: 18–22, 1971.

11. McQuillan, L. M., Lopec, C. A., and Vibal, J. R., Evaluation of EEG and clinical changes associated with Pavabid therapy in chronic brain syndrome. *Curr. Ther. Res.* 16: 49–58, 1974.

12. Branconnier, R. J., and Cole, J. O., Effects of chronic papaverine administration on mild senile organic brain syndrome. *J. Amer. Geriatrics Soc.* 25: 458–462, 1977.

13. Bazo, A. J., An ergot alkaloid preparation (hydergine) versus papaverine in treating common complaints of the aged: Doubleblind study. *J. Amer. Geriatrics Soc.* 21: 63–71, 1973.

14. Rosen, H. J., Mental decline in the elderly: Pharmacotherapy (ergot alkaloids versus papaverine). *J. Amer. Geriatrics Soc.* 23: 169–174, 1975.

15. Branconnier, R., and Cole, J. O., Senile dementia and drug therapy. In *The Aging Brain and Senile Dementia: Advances in Behavioral Biology,* Vol. 23, ed. by K. Nandy and I. Sherwin, Plenum Press, New York, 1977, pp. 271–283.

16. Judge, T. G., and Urquihart, A., Naftidrofuryl—a double blind crossover study in the elderly. *Curr. Med. Res. Opinion* 1: 166–172, 1972.

17. Bouvier, J. B., Passeron, O., and Chapin, M. P., Psychometric study of Praxilene. *J. Intern. Med. Res.* 2: 59–65, 1974.
18. Gerin, J., Double-blind trial of naftidrofuryl in the treatment of cerebral arteriosclerosis. *Brit. J. Clin. Pract.* 28: 177–178, 1974.
19. Cox, J. R., Double-blind evaluation of naftidrofuryl in treating elderly confused, hospitalized patients. *Geront. Clin.* (Basel) 17: 160–167, 1975.
20. Brodie, N. H., A double-blind trial of naftidrofuryl in treating confused elderly patients in general practice. *Practitioner* 218: 274–279, 1977.
21. Jacobs, E. A., Winter, P. M., Alvis, H. J., et al., Hyperoxygenation effects on cognitive functioning in the aged. *New England J. Med.* 281: 753–757, 1969.
22. Ben-Yishay, Y., Diller, L., Warga, C., et al., The alleviation of cognitive and functional impairments in senility by hyperbaric oxygenation combined with systematic cuing. In W. G. Trapp, E. W. Bannister, A. J. Davison, et al. (eds.), *Fifth International Hyperbaric Conference,* Simon Fraser University Press, Burnaby, Canada, 1974, Vol. 1, pp. 424–431.
23. Boyle, E., Aparicio, A., Canosa, F., et al., Hyperbaric oxygen and acetazolamide in the treatment of senile cognitive functions. In W. G. Trapp, E. W. Bannister, A. J. Davison, et al. (eds.), *Fifth International Hyperbaric Conference,* Burnaby, Canada, Simon Fraser University Press, 1974, Vol. 1, pp. 432–438.
24. Edwards, A. E., and Hart, G. M., Hyperbaric oxygenation and the cognitive functioning of the aged. *J. Amer. Geriatrics Soc.* 22: 376–379, 1974.
25. Imai, Y., Hyperbaric oxygen (OHP) therapy in memory disturbances. In W. G. Trapp, E. W. Bannister, A. J. Davison, et al. (eds.), *Fifth International Hyperbaric Conference,* Burnaby, Canada, Simon Fraser University Press, 1974, Vol. 1, pp. 402–408.
26. Jacobs, E. A., Alvis, H. J., and Small, S. M., Hyperoxygenation: A central nervous system activator? *J. Geriatric Psychiat.* 5: 107–121, 1972.
27. Thompson, L. W., Davis, G. C., Obrist, W., et al., Effects of hyperbaric oxygen on behavioral and physiological measures in elderly demented patients. *J. Geront.* 31: 23–28, 1976.
28. Raskin, A., Gershon, S., Crook, T. H., Sathananthan, G., and Ferris, S., The effects of hyperbaric and normobaric oxygen on cognitive impairment in the elderly. *Arch. Gen. Psychiat.* 35: 50–56, 1978.
29. Ellis, Janius, Pure oxygen inhalation a curative. *Moneysworth,* January 1977.
30. Rossi, Rosalind, Pressured oxygen a cure for senility? *Moneysworth,* May 1979, p. 4.
31. Aslan, A., Procaine therapy in old age and other disorders (novocaine factor H3). *Geront. Clin.* 3: 148, 1960.
32. Aslan, A., Therapeutics of old age—the action of procaine. In *Medical and*

Clinical Aspects of Aging, ed. by H. T. Blumenthal, Columbia University Press, New York, 1962, pp. 279–292.

33. Aslan, A., Theoretical and practical aspects of chemotherapeutic techniques in the retardation of the aging process. In *Theoretical Aspects of Aging,* ed. by M. Rockstein, Academic Press, New York, 1974, pp. 177–186.

34. Sakalis, G., Gershon, S., and Shopsin, B., A trial of Gerovital-H3 in depression during senility. *Curr. Ther. Res.* 16: 59–63, 1974.

35. Cohen, S., and Ditman, K. S., Gerovital-H3 in the treatment of the depressed aging patient. *Psychosomatics* 15: 15–19, 1974.

36. Zung, W. K., Gianturco, D., Pfeiffer, E., Wang, H. S., Whanger, A., Bride, T. P., and Potkin, S. G., Pharmacology of depression in the aged: Evaluation of Gerovital H-3 as an antidepressant drug. *Psychosomatics* 15: 127–131, 1974.

37. *Physician's Desk Reference, 33rd Edition, 1979,* Medical Economics Company, a division of Litton Industries, Inc., Oradell, N.J., 1979, pp. 788, 935.

38. Crook, T., Central-nervous-system stimulants: Appraisal of use in geropsychiatric patients. *J. Amer. Geriatrics Soc.* 27: 476–477, 1979.

39. Tecce, J. J., and Cole, J. O., Amphetamine effects in man: Paradoxical drowsiness and lowered brain activity (CNV). *Science* 85: 451–453, 1974.

40. Crook, T., Ferris, S., Sathananthan, G., Raskin, A., and Gershon, S., The effect of methylphenidate on test performance in the cognitively impaired aged. *Psychopharmacology* 52: 251–255, 1977.

41. Prien, R. F., Chemotherapy in chronic organic brain syndrome—a review of the literature. *Psychopharmacol. Bull.* 9: 5–20, 1973.

42. Reisberg, B., Ferris, S., and Gershon, S., Psychopharmacologic aspects of cognitive research in the elderly: Some current perspectives. *Interdisciplinary Topics in Gerontology,* ed. by W. Meier-Ruge and H. von Hahn, Vol. 15, *CNS Aging and Its Neuropharmacology: Experimental and Clinical Aspects,* S. Karger, Basel, 1979, pp. 132–152.

43. Dimond, S. J., and Brouwers, E. Y. M., Increase in the power of human memory in normal man through the use of drugs. *Psychopharmacology* 49: 307–309, 1976.

44. Mindus, P., Cronholm, B., Levander, S. E., and Schalling, D., Piracetam-induced improvement of mental performance: A controlled study on normally aging individuals. *Acta Psychiat. Scand.* 54: 150–160, 1976.

45. Stegink, A. J., The clinical use of piracetam, a new nootropic drug: The treatment of symptoms of senile involution. *Arzneimittel-Forsch.* 22: 975–977, 1972.

46. Abuzzahab, F. S., Merwin, G. E., Zimmerman, R. L., and Sherman, M. C., A doubleblind investigation of piracetam (Nootropil) versus

placebo in the memory of geriatric inpatients. *Psychopharmacol. Bull.* 14(1): 23–25, Jan. 1978.

47. Trabant, R., Poljakovic, Z., and Trabant, D., Zur Wirkung von Piracetam auf das hirnorganische Psychsyndrom bei zerebrovaskularer Insuffizienze: Ergebnis einer Doppelblindstudie bei 40 Fallen. *Therapie Gegnw.* 116: 1504–1521, 1977.

48. Niall, H. D., and Tregear, G. W., Peptide-hormone analogues. *New England J. Med.* 301: 940–941, 1979.

49. De Wied, D., Influence of anterior pituitary on avoidance learning and escape behavior. *Amer. J. Physiol.* 207: 255–259, 1964.

50. De Wied, D., Inhibitory effect of ACTH and related peptides on extinction of conditioned avoidance behavior in rats. *Proc. Soc. Exp. Biol. Med.* 122: 28–32, 1966.

51. De Wied, D., and Bohus, B., Long-term and short-term effect on retention of a conditioned avoidance response in rats by treatment respectively with long-acting pitressin or α-MSH. *Nature* (London) 212: 1484–1486, 1966.

52. Weiss, J. M., McEwen, B. S., Silva, M. T., and Kalkut, M., Pituitary-adrenal alterations and fear responding. *Amer. J. Physiol.* 218: 864–868, 1970.

53. Otsuka, H., and Inouye, K., Synthesis of peptides related to the N-terminal structure of corticotropin: II. The synthesis of L-histidyl-L-phenylalanyl-L-arginyl-L-tryptophan, the smallest peptide exhibiting the melanocyte stimulating and lipolytic activities. *Bull. Chem. Soc. Jap.* 37: 1465–1471, 1964.

54. Greven, H. N., and De Wied, D., The influence of peptides derived from ACTH on performance structure activity studies. In *Progress in Brain Research,* Vol. 39, *Drug Effects on Neuroendocrine Regulation,* ed. by E. Zimmerman, W. H. Gispen, B. H. Marks, and D. De Wied, Elsevier, Amsterdam, 1973, pp. 429–442.

55. Ferris, S. H., Sathananthan, G., Gershon, S., Clark, C., and Moshinsky, J., Cognitive effects of ACTH-4-10 in the elderly. *Pharmacol. Biochem. Behav.* 5: Suppl. 1, 73–78, 1976.

56. Will, J. C., Abuzzahab, F. S., and Zimmerman, R. L., The effects of ACTH 4-10 versus placebo in the memory of symptomatic geriatric volunteers. *Psychopharmacol. Bull.* 14(1): 25–27, Jan. 1978.

57. Branconnier, R. D. J., Cole, J. O., and Gardos, G., ACTH 4-10 in the amelioration of neuropsychological symptomatology associated with senile organic brain syndrom. *Psychopharmacol. Bull.* 14: (1): 27–30, 1978.

58. Bohus, B., Greidanus, T. V. W., and De Wied, D., Behavioral and endocrine responses of rats with hereditary hypothalamic diabetes insipidus (Brattleboro strain). *Physiol. Behav.* 14: 609–615, 1975.

59. Greidanus, T. V. W., Dogterom, J., and De Wied, D., Intraventricular

administration of antivasopressin serum inhibits memory consolidation in rats. *Life Sci.* 16: 637–644, 1975.

60. Lande, S., Flexner, J. B., and Flexner, L. B., Effect of corticotropin and desglycinamide⁹-lysine vasopressin on suppression of memory by puromycin. *Proc. Nat. Acad. Sci. U.S.A.* 69: 558–560, 1972.

61. Oliveros, J. C., Jandali, M. K., Timsit-Berthier, M., Remy, R., Benghezal, A., Audibert, A., and Moeslen, J. M., Vasopressin in amnesia. *Lancet* i: 42, 1978.

62. Legros, J. J., Gilot, P., Seron, X., Claessen, J., Adam, A., Moeglen, J. M., Audibert, A., and Berchier, P., Influence of vasopressin on learning and memory. *Lancet* i: 41–42, 1978.

63. Rigter, H., Attentuation of amnesia in rats by systemically administered enkephaline. *Science* 200: 83–85, 1978.

64. Ferris, S. H., Sathananthan, G., Reisberg, B., and Gershon, S., Long-term choline treatment of memory-impaired elderly patients. *Science* 205, 1039–1040, 1979.

65. "Psychopharmacology of Neurotransmitter Systems in Aging." Awarded by the National Institute of Mental Health, Grant #1 RO 1 MH 29590—01 CPP.

66. Hirsch, M. J., Growden, J. H., and Wurtman, R. J., Relations between dietary choline or lecithin intake, serum choline levels and various metabolic indices. *Metabolism* 27: 953–960, 1978.

67. Etienne, P., Gauthier, S., Dastoor, D., Collier, B., and Ratner, J., Lecithin in Alzheimer's disease. *Lancet* i: 508, 1978.

68. Davis, K. L., Mohs, R. C., and Tinklenberg, J. R., Enhancement of memory by physostigmine. *New England J. Med.,* Oct. 25, 1979, p. 940.

69. Peters, B. H., and Levin, H. S., Effects of physostigmine and lecithin on memory in Alzheimer's disease. *Ann. Neurol.* 6: 219–221, 1979.

Chapter 8

Treating Senility: Psychotherapy and Counseling

THE HISTORY OF psychotherapeutic approaches to the treatment of Alzheimer's disease has, not surprisingly, in many ways paralleled the story of our emerging interest and understanding of the disease itself.

We have already mentioned Western medicine's traditional concentration on the alleviation of acute illness. In terms of the historical forces shaping the development of medicine as an art, a science, and a profession, this emphasis is not surprising.

Acute illnesses, by definition, tend to resolve, for better or worse, in a relatively short period of time. In most instances, because of the body's adequate protective and homeostatic mechanisms, acute illnesses improve or disappear entirely. This process inherently works in favor of *any* treatment intervention strategies. If the treatments do not result in actual harm, then the outcome tends to be relatively encouraging. The net result is optimism on the part of the patient, the originator of the therapeutic strategy, and the practitioner. The optimism, understandably, has a salutary effect upon the entire profession.

Chronic or morbid illnesses, such as arthritis, cancer, or senility, are much more difficult to relieve. These conditions tend to worsen unless a dramatically effective cure is found. Even when effective interventions are developed, such as the ones which are currently

146

available for many forms of cancer, the condition still tends to progress, albeit at a slower pace. Demonstrating the relative efficacy of such interventions takes many years. Hence practitioners and applied researchers, quite naturally, find the alleviation of acute illness more rewarding in many ways and therefore focus their attentions and investigations in that direction.

Similarly, traditional psychotherapy has focused upon relatively acute and "curable" conditions. An ideal candidate for classical psychoanalysis was young, verbal, intelligent, and capable of "insight." The latter was seen as essential for any eventual therapeutic success. "A youthful mind, in terms of actual years or a certain elasticity of functioning, is essential. In general, treatment proceeds more quickly to an effective result when the patient is in his 20's or 30's."[1]

Obviously, persons with Alzheimer's disease are neither young nor eloquent nor particularly noted for their intellectual insightfulness. "Insight" was traditionally considered necessary for therapeutic candidates to "work through" their "transference" feelings for the therapist arising from their previous "relationships with significant others."

Some of these supposed deficiencies of persons with Alzheimer's disease, from a traditional psychoanalytic perspective, may also be said to apply to schizophrenics. Nevertheless, some traditionally trained analysts eventually did turn their attention toward psychotherapeutic treatment of younger schizophrenics. In the 1920s Harry Stack Sullivan may have been the first to report on therapeutic approaches to these severely disturbed patients. Frieda Fromm-Reichmann reported upon her psychotherapeutic treatment of schizophrenics in the following decade. Other, currently well-known therapists subsequently took up the cause, among them Otto Will and R. D. Laing.

However, even after various psychotherapeutic modalities were widely applied to even the most regressed schizophrenic patients, the elderly in general continued to be viewed as too "rigid" and "set in their ways" for such intervention.

The senile were particularly set apart, and this separation permitted psychiatrists and other psychotherapists to ignore them successfully. In terms of the psychiatric nomenclature, persons with what we now know to be Alzheimer's disease are classified as suffering from "chronic organic brain syndrome."[2,3] The conceptualization of the characteristics of the "senile dementia" subtype of organic brain syndrome is instructive. The 1968 edition of the *Diagnostic and Statistical Manual of Mental Disorders,* containing psychiatrists' classification guidelines, stated, by way of description, "even mild cases will manifest some evidence of organic brain syndrome: self-centeredness, difficulty in assimilating new experiences, and childish emotionality."[3]

This description may be viewed as pejorative. It may have represented an unconscious rationalization on the part of American psychiatrists for their shameful neglect of this numerically large patient population, often in direct custody of the psychiatric profession. There is no basis for thinking of the senile as being any more self-centered than the rest of us. The statement that they have "difficulty in assimilating new experiences" is more accurate but probably self-serving. It may have been used to rationalize the psychotherapeutic and general professional neglect of these patients. Finally, accusing the senile of "childish emotionality" is probably inaccurate, and curiously imprecise for psychiatric terminology. Senile persons are often anxious; they often manifest denial; they sometimes become agitated or psychotic. All of these real emotional problems frequently experienced by the senile are easily recognized by psychiatrists and fall well within their professional and therapeutic domain. Referring to "childish emotionality" needlessly confuses the young with the old, and adds little or nothing by way of meaningful psychiatric description. Finally, "self-centeredness" and "childish emotionality" are not described characteristics of any of the other numerous forms of "organic brain syndrome." These are defined, more accurately, in the same diagnostic guide as "disorders manifested by the following symptoms: (a) impairment of orientation; (b) impairment of memory; (c) impairment of all intellectual functions, such as comprehension, calculation, knowledge, learning, etc.; (d) impairment of judgment; and (e) lability and shallowness of affect."* This description of the organic brain syndromes in general—which include a wide variety of disorders in which there is identifiable damage to the brain, from brain damage due to alcohol or other toxins to brain tumors—certainly describes senility more accurately than the more specific description offered in this same authoritative diagnostic manual.

As psychotherapy became progressively more eclectic, even the elderly, in nontraditional settings, came to be considered suitable can-

---

* "Affect" is psychiatric terminology for the expression of one's emotions. A "labile affect" is a rapidly varying emotional state. For example, if one begins a conversation cheerfully and starts crying a few moments later for no apparent reason, then one may be described as displaying "lability of affect." A "shallow affect" is a general paucity of emotional responsivity.

didates. During the year of 1974–75, I treated a 67-year-old widow psychotherapeutically, under supervision, within a psychiatric residency training program. My supervisor did not object to my working with a woman of that age. Neither was my supervisor taken aback when my patient, now 68, met an 82-year-old widower, and the couple sought out my services for sex counseling and therapy! Clearly, the idea that age itself precluded emotional growth was being seriously challenged in the 1970s. But what of psychotherapy for Alzheimer's disease victims?

The most widely known psychotherapeutic intervention which has been said to be of specific value in the treatment of senility is a technique known as "Reality Orientation." It is an ostensibly humanistic approach which consists of constant reorienting of the dementia-phase individual. Patients are continually reminded of the date, their surroundings, the time of year, their identity, etc. Proponents of this technique claim it actually restores patients to health.[4]

Unfortunately, there is no objective evidence that it does more than give families and health personnel the illusion that if only they work long enough and sufficiently diligently at this simple technique, they can do something positive to improve the patient's status. It actually appears to be little more than a sensible, scientific-sounding modern ritual. There are positive components to the treatment, however. Senile persons continue to require human contact just as the rest of us do. Challenging their fantasies or attempting to educate and continually reeducate demented persons is probably of no value. However, befriending, communicating with, and comforting the senile is always appropriate.

In the dementia phase, and in the earlier confused and forgetfulness stages, relatives often believe that the disease process can be arrested, or at least treated, "if only they were interested in more things," or "if only they exercised more," or "if only they *used* their minds more." These beliefs are based upon several fallacies. One is that if people don't use their minds properly, then they will decay; another is that brain failure is the result of inactive minds and bodies.[5]

Sadly, many patients develop Alzheimer's disease even though they do not retire. Patients have taken up jogging and achieved better physical health than at any time during their adult lives without apparently altering the inexorable progress of the disease. There is no evidence whatsoever that the disease occurs more or less frequently, or at a different age, among persons who are laborers as opposed to professors; among those who retire as opposed to those who continue to work; among introverts as opposed to extroverts, etc.

Nevertheless, on the basis of these folk beliefs, spouses and other relatives frequently attempt to push the confused- or demented-phase person to "do more." These exhortations and demands provoke anxiety and resentment on the part of patients, who are genuinely no longer capable of meeting the demands of their previous range of activities. Patients become seemingly more withdrawn because the psychic demands of their more circumscribed activities are at, or near, the limits of their current capacities, given their reduced intellectual skills. Indeed, clinicians frequently observe a reduction in anxiety and seeming improvement when a confused-phase patient gets a companion to assist with newly perplexing tasks, such as selecting a new seasonal wardrobe.

Hence a sensible, and truly humanitarian, approach to care would be to provide senile persons with the support which they require, depending upon their current capacities. Attempts to exceed their capabilities should probably be discouraged. Similarly, privacy should be respected. There is probably no harm in the seemingly introverted reveries of the senile person. Just as for other human beings, a genuinely humanistic approach is one which aids in meeting a person's needs, desires, and aspirations and which respects the person's right to eschew that which, for whatever reason, he or she would prefer not to face.

Other systematic approaches in addition to Reality Orientation have recently been applied to the treatment of Alzheimer's patients. One technique is called "Cognitive Training" or "CT." This consists of several memory training sessions which are generally given by a trained therapist on an individual basis.

Mnemonic tools which assist in recalling lists, speeches, poems, etc., have been known since antiquity. They consist of associative devices which can be used to connect otherwise unrelated material. One of the best known is the verse for remembering the number of days in the months: "Thirty days hath September, April, June, and November," etc. More elaborate mnemonic devices are often based on "the technique of the Roman forum." This ingenious method involves memorizing the location of rooms, furniture, etc., in a large house. If one then wants to memorize a list of unrelated things, one associates each item of the list with a part of the house. Association makes recall less difficult.

Mnemonic devices are undoubtedly invaluable in performing impressive feats of memory. They may also be useful in helping forgetful-phase persons to recall certain important items which they tend to have difficulty remembering, such as clients' names and addresses. Even confused-phase persons may benefit from cognitive training (CT) in coping with their cognitive disability. Dementia-phase individuals are probably too impaired to benefit from CT. Since their primary disability is in remembering recently acquired information, they may forget their training lessons even more quickly than the previously learned material which they are having difficulty retrieving from memory.

Investigators have recently begun to evaluate the usefulness of CT in the treatment of persons with various stages of senile memory impairments. For this approach to be proven of genuine value, it will have to be shown to be superior to the more generalized supportive psychotherapeutic techniques. Although CT has not yet been shown to differ in outcome from supportive psychotherapy, the preliminary evidence is that both approaches are superior to no therapy at all.[6]

At New York University we have begun to explore a different, less direct modality of therapy for confused- and dementia-phase persons—family treatment. We have begun group sessions in which either spouses or children who are intimately involved in caring for an impaired individual are able to ventilate their fears and frustrations. Some interesting generalizations have emerged from this preliminary work. Most of the spouses who seek out therapeutic assistance in caring for a senile person appear to be men. This ratio is in contrast to the overall sex ratio of spouses of our clinic patients. Women, who tend to remain healthier and to live longer, predominate overall. Why, then, do more men seek therapy?

The explanation appears to be that men in our society have more difficulty assuming a supportive and caring role than do women. The skills—both technical and emotional—which are learned in raising a family appear to be useful once again at the opposite end of life's spectrum. Men are frequently overwhelmed when confronted with an increasingly helpless spouse whom they are ill prepared to care for. Their confusion and sense of helplessness may find expression as anger. The latter is the dominant emotion expressed by the participants in our spouses' supportive therapy groups.

Children express very different interests and emotions in group and in individual counseling settings. Their major concern is often the future course of their impaired parent's condition. Another anxiety, which is probably more often feared than articulated, centers on heredito-familial aspects of the condition. Children are understandably fearful lest a similar fate becloud their latter years. This fear often brings children to query their physicians and/or their counselors on matters of prevention. Offspring who are responsible for caring for an impaired parent also express very realistic concerns in connection with such practical issues as obtaining assistance in caring for their parents, deciding when it is appropriate for them to consider institutionalization, and deciding upon an appropriate institution at the proper time.

A counselor-therapist is obligated to address these pragmatic issues in as informative and helpful a manner as possible. Concise answers to each of these frequently asked questions can be formulated based upon currently available knowledge and supports.

Q. What will happen to my relative in the future?

A. At the present time only a limited amount of information concerning the prognosis of your relative's condition is available. Part of the reason for this is that scientists and physicians have turned their attention to the study of senility and age-associated memory loss only over the past several years. Since memory loss is a very gradual process, there has not been sufficient time for doctors to get a true picture of the long-term course of the condition.

From what we currently know, it is certainly possible that your relative will get worse. How quickly this happens varies from one person to another. Some people appear to deteriorate from the point where their memories are satisfactory to the point where they are incapable of functioning on their own over a period of only a few years. Other people show the same deterioration over the course of more than a decade. At present we do not really know why some people get worse rapidly and others deteriorate much more slowly.

It is also possible that your relative will not get noticeably worse in the next year or two. Many of the people whom we examine carefully on follow-up visits after 12 months are no worse than they were a year before. Some people actually seem to improve somewhat over the course of a year. Even severely impaired people do not necessarily get worse quickly. One severely impaired woman whom we carefully evaluated and then carefully reevaluated two years later did about the same on most of our tests on both occasions. Persons with very mild or mild impairment may actually get better.

Unfortunately, we have not yet identified the characteristics which would indicate a relatively good or a relatively poor prognosis. Hence, until more knowledge becomes available, I would suggest that a sensible approach to your relative's condition would be to hope for the best and prepare yourself for the worst.

Q. How can I be certain my relative has been properly diagnosed? How can I be certain my relative really has senility, or Alzheimer's disease as you call it, and not some other condition?

A. The diagnosis of Alzheimer's disease is what physicians call a "diagnosis of exclusion." By this they mean that a very wide variety of other possible causes must be ruled out for your doctor to be certain that the diagnosis is correct. Even though a very long list of other conditions can cause the symptoms which your relative has, a skilled and experienced physician can, in fact, arrive at an accurate diagnosis with some certainty. In most cases, the diagnosis can be determined after the appropriate diagnostic tests have been performed, in only one or two visits. Naturally, at times the diagnosis may be more complicated. Hence the real problem is often finding a skilled and experienced physician to arrive at the diagnosis. This problem is considerably complicated by the fact that conditions which fall within the realms of many different medical specialties must be ruled out for a proper diagnosis to be made. One of the most important conditions to be considered is serious depression. This condition frequently causes similar symptoms and can appear very similar to senility. Furthermore, depression is also seen more frequently in the elderly. Only psychiatrists are expert at diagnosing depression, and many other physicians have difficulty recognizing this condition, particularly since there are no laboratory tests which can be used to assist in making the diagnosis.

Other possible causes of senility which require consideration fall within an internist's area of primary expertise. These include various possible hormonal causes of senility, as well as various other less frequent medical causes such as kidney or liver problems.

Finally, conditions such as Parkinsonism, which may also mimic senility, are most easily recognized by neurologists. Neurologists may also be relatively expert in diagnosing various brain conditions which can mimic senility.

The best initial approach for relatives is probably for them to find a physician who specializes in treating either Alzheimer's disease itself or the elderly in general, from one of these three medical disciplines mentioned, i.e., a geriatric psychiatrist, or an internist specializing in geriatrics, or a geriatric neurologist.

There are many ways in which such a physician can be located. One excellent approach is to contact the local Alzheimer's disease society if one exists in your area. A list of such societies can be found in Table 8–1. Since all of these societies have been established very recently and new societies are being formed very rapidly, it is possible that a society will exist in your area even if it is not listed in Table 8–1. I would recommend your contacting the society nearest to you and asking them for more specific information regarding services in your area.

An association consisting of psychiatrists who specialize in the treatment of the elderly has recently been formed. This group is known as the American Association for Geriatric Psychiatry (AAGP). Beginning in the year 1979–80, they made available a Membership Listing. This consists of information on over 300 psychiatrists in the United States and Canada. Listings are also included of geriatric psychiatrists from seven countries outside of North America. In addition to providing the names and addresses of geriatric psychiatrists, listed according to region, the AAGP Membership Listing provides information regarding the activities of each of the members. The Membership Listing can be obtained by writing to:

American Association for Geriatric Psychiatry
230 North Michigan Avenue, Suite 2400
Chicago, Ill. 60601

Physicians from various specialties who are particularly interested in the treatment of the elderly are members of the American Geriatrics Society. Information regarding members can be obtained by contacting:

American Geriatrics Society
10 Columbus Circle, Room 1470
New York, N.Y. 10019

Another organization with a diverse membership which includes physicians from many different specialties is the Gerontological Society. This organization, which is devoted to research on aging, has a Clinical Medicine Section which is primarily for its physician members. Information regarding society members can be obtained by contacting:

Gerontological Society
1835 K Street, N.W.
Washington, D.C. 20006

TABLE 8-1. Alzheimer's Disease Societies

Bronx, New York
Yeshiva University
Alzheimer Project
Bronx, N.Y.

Columbus, Ohio
National Alzheimer Foundation
4950 Olde Coventry Rd. West
Columbus, Ohio 43227
Attn: Ms. Nancy Schlegal, R.N.

Englewood Cliffs, New Jersey
Alzheimer's Disease Society
560 Sylvan Avenue
Englewood Cliffs, N.J. 07632

Minneapolis, Minnesota
R.E.A.C.H.
c/o Mental Health Association of Minnesota
4510 West 77th Street
Minneapolis, Minn. 55435

New York, New York
Alzheimer's Disease Society
32 Broadway
New York, N.Y. 10004
Attn: Mr. Lonnie E. Wollin, Sec. Treas.

Philadelphia, Pennsylvania
Pennsylvania School of Medicine
Alzheimer Project
Philadelphia, Pa.

San Francisco, California
Family Survival Project
Mental Health Foundation of San Francisco
1745 Van Ness Avenue
San Francisco, Calif. 94109

Seattle, Washington
A.S.I.S.T. (Alzheimer's Support Information and Services Team)
c/o Department of Psychiatry and Behavioral Sciences
RP-10
University of Washington
Seattle, Wash. 98195

Toronto, Canada
Société Alzheimer Society
2 Surrey Place
Toronto, Ontario M5S 2C2
Canada

In those instances where the above services have not enabled you to contact a local physician with expertise in the diagnosis of Alzheimer's disease and other causes of memory impairment in the elderly, more general approaches may be taken in order to locate the best possible physician. You can contact your county medical society and request assistance, or you can contact your local hospital directly.

Q. What kind of evaluation should my doctor do? What tests should the doctor order?

A. This will vary widely depending upon the individual physician, your relative's background, and availability of economic resources. In general, the most comprehensive diagnostic workup is much less costly in terms of both time and money than even a brief period of hospitalization. However, third parties, such as government and private medical insurance agencies, often reimburse hospital costs more readily than outpatient treatment expenses. Hence the cost to you of a complete diagnostic workup may seem relatively large in comparison to hospital costs, since you are not being reimbursed.

Your doctor will certainly obtain a complete medical history. Many aspects of your relative's medical background are of particular relevance to his or her thinking problem. For example, conditions resulting from diabetes, gland disturbances, and liver, kidney, and heart problems can all be contributing to the thinking disturbance. Your doctor will also want to find out whether your relative has a history of mental disturbances. This is absolutely essential, since many of your relative's symptoms can be caused by such conditions.

The physician should also obtain some information regarding your relative's social and occupational background. This can have direct as well as indirect relevance. Obviously, if your relative never had the opportunity to attend primary school, he or she will perform very differently from a retired mathematics teacher on a test of calculating ability. These factors need to be taken into consideration. Also, chronic exposure to a very wide variety of toxic chemicals at work and/or elsewhere in one's surroundings can result in symptoms very similar to those of senility. Your doctor will want to determine whether there is any likelihood that your relative has suffered from such exposure.

Of course, your relative will then receive a complete physical examination. This should include a neurological examination and a psychiatric examination, sometimes referred to as a "mental status examination."

After the above steps have been completed, the necessary tests will be ordered. Routine blood tests will be done. These can give your doctor an indication as to whether your relative has medically significant liver problems, kidney problems, etc. A urinanalysis will assist in these evaluations.

Beyond these routine tests, your doctor may order certain special procedures in evaluating your relative's thinking problem. These include an electroencephalogram and a brain scan. An electroencephalogram is a brain wave recording. It is done by placing wires over the scalp surface. Sometimes pads or a special paste is used to assist in the conduction of the electricity from the brain. The procedure usually does not require any needles, and there is no pain either during or after the recording. Your relative simply must sit quietly in a chair. The presence of abnormal brain waves may indicate the presence of brain injury. This can be the result of a fall, a stroke, a tumor, or some other condition.

A brain scan is a picture of the substance of the brain. The older kind of brain scan requires an injection of a radioactive substance into the arm in order to get a picture of the brain. The more modern kind of brain scan is called a "CT scan," a "CAT scan," or, in its long form, a "computer-assisted tomographic scan." It does not require any injections, and there is no pain. This amazing new device enables physicians to get a clear picture of your relative's brain. This is accomplished by using a computer to reconstruct brain "slices" mathematically from X-ray images. The pictures of the brain substance which are produced can tell your doctor whether there is visible injury to the substance of the brain. The pictures also reveal the presence of brain shrinkage and decay and can reveal the presence of past strokes. These pictures can be valuable in enabling your doctor to arrive at a final diagnosis. A CT scan usually costs approximately $200. The radiation exposure is comparable to that of a chest X-ray. Brain tissue, for various reasons, is not very sensitive to X-ray damage, particularly in older people. Hence a CT scan is a valuable diagnostic aid which causes essentially no discomfort to the patient and is not known to be associated with any significant risks.

Q. If I follow your advice and consult an expert physician, and the doctor, after a complete evaluation, confirms the diagnosis of senility, or Alzheimer's disease as you call it, is there anything further which can be done to help my relative, or is the situation hopeless?

A. At the present time, as you probably are aware, we do not have any dramatic cures. Neither do we have any substances which can dramatically reverse the condition. However, there are substances, which your doctor can prescribe, which may be useful in decreasing the rate at which the condition would ordinarily worsen. Naturally, these substances are useful only if your relative continues to take them regularly over a period of years. It is important that you keep in mind that senility is a chronic condition which requires long-term treatment.

Another area in which your physician may be of help is in relieving some of the emotional disturbances, in the patient and those closest to him, which may occur over the course of your relative's illness. Finally, your physician should be in a position to advise you on specific strategies for coping with your relative's impairment.

Q. Speaking of coping, my relative has begun to get lost and wander away from home. What am I to do?

A. One thing which can be done is to have a double lock installed on the door. This is one which can be locked from the inside as well as from without. Naturally, for safety purposes, you will want to have a key available nearby at all times. This may be hung up at a convenient location. Relatives who are that confused will not remember where the key has been placed, and when they absent-mindedly go to the door, they will find it locked.

Another precaution which you will probably wish to take immediately is to sew identification labels into your relative's clothing. You might also wish to consider identification jewelry. Since necklaces are frequently removed, a wrist bracelet with a lock is often best.

If your relative has already wandered off on more than one occasion and you are particularly worried, I would also consider purchasing an electronic signaling device. These can be placed in a pocket or on a necklace. If your relative wanders off, then a receiver can be used to locate him or her by homing in on the signal. The local police are often very helpful not only in assisting in locating a relative in a time of crisis but also in providing useful suggestions regarding ways of watching and keeping track of a relative so as to avoid a crisis.

Q. Looking after my relative is a full-time job, 24 hours a day, day and night. I need some relief, at least part of the time. Where can I get help?

A. This is one of the most common problems which relatives of senile persons face. Homemakers are available through several sources. One source which you can contact is:

> National Council for Homemakers
> Home Health Aide Services
> 1790 Broadway
> New York, N.Y. 10019

The major problem is usually not finding a homemaker, however; it is finding some means of paying for such assistance in a home setting. The medical assistance program for elderly persons is known as "Medicare." All elderly persons who have passed a specified minimum age are eligible for Medicare assistance. Although Medicare is primarily a federal program, services vary somewhat from state to state. Medicare ordinarily will not reimburse the cost of homemaker services, even when they are considered to be medically necessary. You can contact your local Social Security office to determine the precise Medicare regulations in your state. Medicaid, the assistance program for the financially indigent, sometimes does reimburse the costs of a homemaker whom your physician believes is medically necessary. Medicaid is a federally assisted, state-run medical assistance program. Hence you will have to contact your local Medicaid office to determine the regulations and requirements in your state.

Unfortunately, needed assistance is often unavailable for homemaker services. "Although keeping a patient in a nursing home is far more expensive, Federal aid encourages institutionalization. Medicaid, for example, covers the entire costs of nursing-home care for indigent patients; in 1977, it paid $7.6 billion in such costs, but only $179 million for home health programs."[7]

Under the present circumstances, less expensive companion services should be considered. Many families find that the part-time services of an enthusiastic young person, often a student, are inexpensive and relatively precious. Day care and community programs for the elderly may also provide assistance.

Q. When should I begin to consider a nursing home?

A. I recommend that long-term institutional care be considered earlier rather than later. This is in keeping with my recommendation that you "hope for the best but prepare yourself for the worst." "Earlier consideration" would mean, in this instance, at the time when your relative begins to require frequent assistance and supervision.

There are many different types of nursing homes and residential facilities for the elderly, and choosing the proper environment requires time and effort on the part of the family.

A primary consideration is frequently proximity and accessibility for family visits. This emphasis is no doubt proper. The availability of family presence and emotional support definitely has much to do with the health and well-being of a senile person in an institution. I have no doubt that concerned families actually keep impaired relatives alive.

Other considerations center upon the needs of the senile person. If there is a virtually uncontrollable tendency to wander, then adequate supervision and security are essential. In an urban setting, this may of necessity include an alarm system at all of the exits. Many senile people, particularly those with other health problems, require relatively frequent medical supervision and nursing care. The level of medical and nursing care varies enormously from one institution to another, and a facility with adequate medical and nursing resources must be located.

An additional consideration which is of great importance centers upon the social needs of the senile person. A home should be selected where your relative can establish friendships and relationships, perhaps with persons with similar backgrounds, who are confronting similar illnesses. The facility should also offer a range of group and social activities in which your relative can participate. Human contact is undoubtedly as important to the elderly and the senile as it is to the rest of us.

Financial considerations also dictate advance planning in case institutionalization should become necessary. Old-age institutions are enormously expensive. Accordingly, assistance is nearly always required in meeting the costs of care. Most often this assistance is in the form of public money from either the Medicare or the Medicaid program.

Medicare benefits in nursing homes tend to be extremely limited. Only persons in Medicare-certified homes are eligible for hospitalization coverage. Furthermore, "benefits cover only the first one-hundred days of care; patients must first have been hospitalized; and only persons with conditions certified as requiring 'skilled' nursing care may be covered, and that condition must be related to the illness that caused the initial hospitalization."[8] These federal regulations and requirements become quite complex. Unfortunately, the details also change as amendments are added from time to time. I strongly urge everyone to become familiar with the applicable regulations at the appropriate time.

Medicaid benefits are available to financially needy persons regardless of age. For eligible persons, these benefits provide for long-term nursing home care without requiring previous hospitalization. These benefits are a major source of economic support for nursing home care. Unfortunately, "in order to qualify for financial assistance in meeting costs, many states require the older person to be indigent, with no assets of his own. If he owns a house, it may have to be turned over to the state or county. The middle-income patient is often in the dilemma of having too much income to be eligible for assistance, yet not enough to afford care on his own."[9]

In trying to choose an adequate supportive facility, families are, of necessity, placed in the position of trying to find adequate logistical, social, and financial solutions for the problems of their impaired relative. These solutions are often impossible to resolve adequately in a crisis period of a few months; indeed, they often require years of careful investigation and planning.

Q. Should I feel guilty about sending my relative away to an institution?

A. This is a question which relatives invariably ask, and I have seen relatives whose feelings of guilt remained acute years after their senile relative had ceased being able to function in a community setting even with the most constant support which could reasonably be provided and had gone into a home.

There are no perfect answers. All elderly people generally fear nursing homes and old-age institutions. The statistics provide ample evidence to justify those fears. One-third of all persons admitted to nursing homes die within the first year. Another third are dead within three years.[9] These statistics are often cited to justify accusations of callousness on the part of relatives. However, they may indicate quite the opposite. It may be that families maintain the frail and the debilitated as long as possible and only surrender their relatives after maintenance of health and well-being has become impossible.

Other statistics may also reflect favorably on the strength and compassion of the family in modern society. According to one survey, over half of the persons in old-age institutions have no close family members.[10] This may indicate that families are indeed supporting their relatives as long as humanly possible.

Guilt feelings over close relatives are natural. However, I would recommend channeling those feelings in specific useful directions. Energy should be expended in finding and providing for the maximum possible level of care. Even more important is ongoing social and emotional support, whether your relative remains at home or enters an institution.

Q. Will the same fate befall me? Will I become senile like my parents? Is senility inherited?

A. Although we are beginning to accumulate preliminary evidence with respect to the role of genetic factors in senility, we really are unsure to what extent heredity contributes to the condition at this time.

Q. Is there anything I can do to prevent it from happening to me?

A. At the present time, scientists and physicians have no information whatsoever on useful prevention measures. The national scientific institutes have recently begun to recognize the importance of the general question of prevention in the reduction of illness. Hence it is possible that eventually the necessary studies will be conducted and physicians will have more to offer in this area.

Q. What exactly are scientists doing in this area? Is there really hope for the future?

A. In the past decade or so, scientists have actually made enormous progress in understanding senility. As you know, we formerly thought of the condition as due to hardening of the arteries, or "arteriosclerosis." We now know that most cases of senility are actually due to a different condition, which we call "Alzheimer's disease." This condition causes characteristic changes in certain parts of the brain. It is also associated with shrinkage of certain parts of the brain. Scientists currently have many theories about the origins of Alzheimer's disease; however, they are still uncertain about its real cause or causes. Scientists and physicians also have many leads as to possibly effective treatments, but these will need to be tested and that will take time.

To properly appreciate the progress which has been made, it is necessary to understand that scientists have learned much more about this condition in the past quarter century than was discovered in all of human history until that time. Medicine is currently undergoing a fascinating and exciting technological revolution in which computers and other modern instruments are being applied to the solution of many basic problems. In the next several years this revolution should help support progress of even greater magnitude. This revolution and its specific applications to the problems of senility are the substance of the following chapter.

Notes

1. Theories of personality and psychopathology: I. Freudian school. In *Modern Synopsis of Comprehensive Textbook of Psychiatry,* ed. by A. M. Freedman, H. I. Kaplan, and B. J. Saddock, Williams & Wilkins Company, Baltimore, 1972, p. 118.
2. *Diagnostic and Statistical Manual of Mental Disorders,* 1st ed., American Psychiatric Association, Washington, D.C., 1952.
3. *Diagnostic and Statistical Manual of Mental Disorders,* 2d ed., American Psychiatric Association, Washington, D.C., 1968.
4. Freese, A. S., Treating the untreatable: The new way to end senility. In *The End of Senility,* Arbor House, New York, 1978, pp. 148–159.
5. Henig, Robin M., Exposing the myth of senility. *New York Times Magazine,* Dec. 3, 1978, p. 158 ff.
6. Yesavage, J. A., Westphal, J., and Rush, L., Combined pharmacological and psychological treatment for senile dementia. Presented at the American Gerontological Society, Washington, D.C., November 1979.
7. Seligman, J., Hager, M., Kirsch, J. and Wilson, C. H., Home care pays off. *Newsweek,* Mar. 10, 1980, p. 107.
8. Manard, B. B., Kart, C. S., and van Gils, D. W. L., *Old-Age Institutions,* Lexington Books, D. C. Heath & Company, Lexington, Mass., p. 34.
9. Butler, R. N.: *Why Survive? Being Old in America.* Harper & Row, New York, 1975, p. 269.
10. Gottesman, L. E., "Nursing Home Performance as Related to Resident Traits, Ownership, Size, and Source of Payment." Philadelphia Geriatric Center, Philadelphia, 1972, mimeographed.

Chapter 9

Future Directions

If you can look into the seeds of time,
And say which grain will grow and which will not,
Speak then to me . . . .

Macbeth, *Act I, Scene 3*

THE PRECEDING CHAPTERS have provided ample and, probably for most readers, surprising evidence of recent progress in our understanding of brain failure in general, and Alzheimer's type brain failure in particular. What kinds of further advances can we realistically hope for in the next few years?

Naturally, serendipitous discoveries and unanticipated complications and frustrations could radically alter any prognostications. However, because science is, after all, a carefully planned enterprise which utilizes and builds upon existing technologies and theoretical conceptualizations, a surprisingly detailed outline of likely future directions is possible. Studies which are currently underway or which are currently being planned will almost certainly increase our understanding of brain failure in every major area. In the next five to ten years we can predict progress in diagnostic and prognostic accuracy with reasonable confidence. New models, which are currently being refined, may accelerate and facilitate the tedious and arduous methods by which therapeutic agents are presently evaluated. With considerably less certainty, we can also reasonably hope for continuing breakthroughs in our basic understanding of the disorder and its ultimate prevention.

164

A formidable array of impressive new technologies are currently being applied to the solution of diagnostic questions in the area of dementia. The most exciting of these technologies have already been mentioned earlier in our story of brain failure. Virtually all utilize a computer to process a vast amount of information which gives us a more accurate picture of brain structure or function. These technologies include computerized axial tomographic scanning of the brain substance ("CT scans," or "CAT scans"), positron emission tomographic imaging of the brain ("PET scans"), and radioisotopic measurements of regional cerebral blood flow (rCBF). Computer analyses have also considerably increased the sophistication of traditional measures of brain electrical activity, such as electroencephalography (EEG). This has resulted in such complex but apparently very useful technologies as quantitative pharmaco-EEG (QPEEG) and "neurometrics."

CT scans are computer-produced pictures of successive "slices" of brain substance. The shading of the picture is determined by the density of the substance visualized. Hence areas of the brain which contain mostly fluid can be distinguished from areas which contain tissue. CT scans also appear to be capable of distinguishing areas of the brain which contain predominately neuronal cells, or "gray matter," from areas of the brain which contain mostly axonal fibers, "white matter."[1]

When first introduced in the mid-1970s, CT scans appeared to hold out considerable promise of enabling clinicians to accurately diagnose senile dementia. Since decay of particular portions of the outermost layers of the brain substance is one of the features observed when autopsies are conducted on the brains of persons with Alzheimer's disease, it was hoped that the extent of brain decay as visualized in CT images would have diagnostic significance. Also, since multi-infarct dementia is characterized by the frequent presence of substantial hemorrhagic areas within the brain—what are referred to at autopsy as "cerebral softenings"—it was hoped that CT scans would be of diagnostic value in this area as well.

In many areas of medicine, and particularly in the field of neurology, CT scans appear to be fulfilling their initial promise. This progress was recognized by the Swedish Academy, which awarded the 1979 Nobel Prize for Physiology and Medicine to the individuals whom they deemed most responsible for the development of this new diagnostic technology. In brain failure, however, CT scans appeared to fall short of their initial promise. A CT scan alone could not reliably distinguish a severely demented person from an unimpaired individual.[2,3,4] Many severely demented people appeared to have normal CT scans.[5] Why?

In Chapter 4, we alluded briefly to some of the reasons why CT scans have not, to date, been of diagnostic significance in and of themselves in senile dementia. One of the most important reasons is the nature of the disease process itself. Alzheimer's disease is characterized primarily by microscopic changes in the substance of the brain. Gross changes, such as overt decay, occur only after the pathological process is well advanced. Analogously, multi-infarct dementia, as the name implies, is marked by the presence of numerous hemorrhagic areas, collectively of significant proportions but individually small in extent.

Many additional problems with CT diagnostic assessment of senile dementia currently exist. For example, the CT pictures are reconstructed from "slices" of the brain (see Figure 9-1). At the present time there are few reliable techniques for positioning the head at identical angles for successive CT imagings. Hence the CT scans, which are actually cross-sectional pictures, are likely to pass through different cross sections and so produce somewhat different pictures not only for different patients but also for the same patient if scans are repeated on subsequent occasions. A variety of ingenious techniques have been proposed as a solution for this problem, particularly for the comparison of successive scans performed on the same patient. For example, some investigators have suggested that a quick-drying plastic cast be made of the head position at the time of the scan and that the patient's head be repositioned in this cast at the time of subsequent scans. Other investigators have suggested the use of videotape playback to reposition the head at the original angle for repeat scanning.[6] Obviously, these "solutions" post logistical problems which might well outweigh their advantages.

Additional problems with attempts which were made initially to utilize CT scans diagnostically in senile dementia included the absence of age-associated norms for comparative purposes and of suitable anatomic landmarks for accurate assessment of the "level" at which the CT scan was taken.

Despite these very real and formidable problems, it does appear that CT scans will be increasingly useful in the diagnosis of dementia in the coming decade. We have already mentioned that groups of CT scans from persons with moderate cognitive impairment appear to

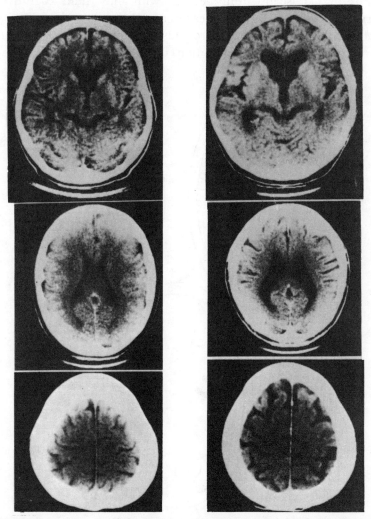

Figure 9.1 Representative CT scans for two ventricular slices (top and middle) and one cortical slice (bottom). Slices on right show more atrophic change than slices on left. The three levels illustrated are (top to bottom): basal ganglia, bodies of the lateral ventricle, and high convexity. These scans were obtained using a GE8800 CT scanner. *Source: De Leon, M. J., Ferris, S. H., George, A. E., Reisberg, B., Kricheff, I. I., and Gershon, S., "Computed tomography evaluations of brain-behavior relationships in senile dementia of the Alzheimer's type,"* in Neurobiology of Aging: Experimental and Clinical Research, *Vol. 1, No. 1, p. 72. Reproduced with permission.*

reveal more expansion of the cerebral ventricles on the average than groups of CT scans from persons with only mild cognitive impairment.[7] Some of the CT measurements that have been utilized to establish these relationships are illustrated in Figure 9–2. The improved resolution of new generations of CT scanners has permitted the

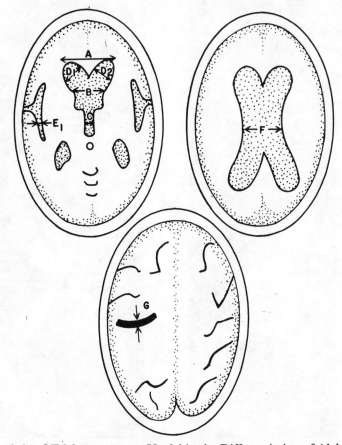

Figure 9.2 CT Measurements Useful in the Differentiation of Alzheimer's Dementia Patients. Illustration of measurements obtained of ventricular and cortical features from CT scans: a) bifrontal span (A); b) bicaudate diameter (B); c) width of the third ventricle (C); d) anterior horns, left and right (D1, D2); e) width of the sylvian Fissures (E1); f) width of the bodies at the waist, (F); and g) sum of the widths of the three largest sulci (G). *Source: De Leon, M. J., Ferris, S. H., George, A. E., Reisberg, B., Kricheff, I. I., and Gershon, S. "Computed tomography evaluation of brain-behavior relationships in senile dementia of the Alzheimer's type,"* in Neurobiology of Aging: Experimental and Clinical Research, *Vol. 1, No. 1, p. 73. Reproduced with permission.*

establishment of these kinds of generalizations. We can expect continued technological advances in scanning techniques over the next decade. We can also expect that information will accumulate on what is normal and what is not for persons of a particular age, sex, head size, and medical history.

Interestingly, it appears possible that investigators will find during the next decade that they had been searching in the wrong areas for CT diagnostic information in senile dementia. As mentioned, until the present, diagnostic studies have concerned themselves with assessing the extent of cortical atrophy and the extent of enlargement of the lateral ventricles of the brain. The enhanced resolution of the current generation of CT scanners may have made very different kinds of diagnostic assessments feasible. For instance, preliminary analyses indicate that the extent of difference in density between the gray and white matter of the cortex may be a diagnostic parameter of significance in Alzheimer's disease.[8] Another recent preliminary finding by our group and others[7,9] is that CT assessment in the vicinity of the *third* ventricle may be an even better index of the extent of cognitive decline in senile dementia than assessments of the lateral ventricles.

The increased resolution of current and future generations of CT scanners should enable clinicians to make analogous progress in the diagnosis of multi-infarct dementia, and in the discrimination and differential diagnosis of such other possible causes of dementia as normal pressure hydrocephalus, Parkinsonism, and affective disorders.

Modern techniques for the assessment of cerebral blood flow—using the inhalation of an inert, radiolabeled gas (generally an isotope of the inert gas xenon, namely xenon 133) and an array of geiger counters joined to a computer, which measures the progress of the radiolabeled substance in the bloodstream through the brain—should also improve our diagnostic assessments in senile dementia (see Figure 9–3). These techniques are currently available at select major medical centers.

It is, of course, anticipated that the physiological changes in Alzheimer's disease and the other causes of dementia will result in predictable and perhaps diagnostically useful changes in cerebral blood flow. Research along these lines has been proceeding for several years.[10,11] One of the most interesting findings, from a diagnostic standpoint, is that the degree of responsivity to a vasodilatory stimulus such as 4 percent carbon dioxide may distinguish the major dementia sub-

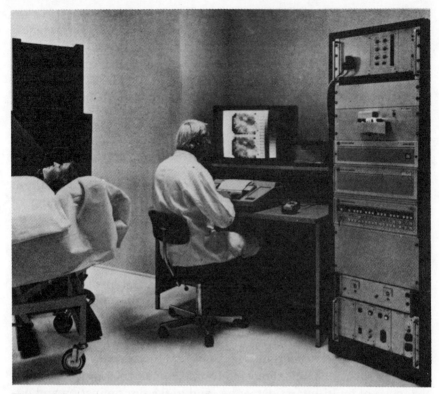

Figure 9.3   Apparatus for Measuring Regional Cerebral Blood Flow (rCBF) Using Radioisotope Inhalation. Brain scan apparatus employed by the authors of the article cited below in their laboratories at Bispebjerg Hospital in Copenhagen and the University of Lund in Sweden is shown during a typical experiment. A few milliliters of saline solution containing xenon 133, a radioactive isotope that emits gamma rays, are injected ino the subject's carotid artery. A battery of 254 externally placed scintillation detectors (located in the box behind the subject's head) then records the arrival and subsequent washout of the radioactive isotope from the cortex during the two minutes after injection. The scintillation data are processed by the computer and are then displayed on the color television screen. *Source: Lassen, N. A., Ingvar, D. H., and Skinhøj, E., "Brain function and blood flow," Scientific American, October 1978, pp. 62–71 (illustration on p. 67).*

types. As mentioned earlier, there is already preliminary evidence that Alzheimer's patients retain the ability to increase cerebral blood flow in response to a vasodilatory stimulus, whereas M.I.D. patients may actually decrease cerebral blood flow in response to the stimulus.[12] Patients with mixed pathology would be expected to fall between the two extremes. If these findings are verified, then rCBF may become a valuable and widely used diagnostic tool in late life dementia.

Another modern technology, which is unlikely to come into routine use in the next decade but which will almost certainly increase our basic understanding of dementia and perhaps improve diagnostic assessments as well, is positron emission tomography, or PET. This technique is analogous in many ways to CT scanning. An important difference is that it enables scientists to obtain a picture of brain function instead of simply providing a structural picture of the brain such as is now widely available using CT scanners. PET requires the injection of a positron-emitting labeled substance into the circulation. The utilization of that substance by the brain is then measured by an array of positron detectors arranged in a semicircle around the head (see Figure 9–4). Because positron-emitting substances decay very rapidly, they must be manufactured shortly before the substance is actually injected into the patient. These constraints of time generally require that PET scans be done in a facility which has a cyclotron that can be used to manufacture the isotope.

One positron-emitting substance which has already been developed is F^{18} deoxyglucose. By injecting this labeled radioisotope of glucose, scientists can obtain a direct assessment of the relative extent to which different brain regions are capable of utilizing glucose for energy and metabolism. Hence the actual viability of brain tissue under varying circumstances can be measured directly.* (See Figure 9–5.)

We have already begun to study glucose utilization in the brains of persons with Alzheimer's disease. Comparisons are being made with control subjects of the same age in an effort to explore the effects of the disease process on energy utilization. Comparisons will be made with the CT pictures, which should provide us with a finer index of the utility and accuracy of the anatomic assessment. Eventually, energy utilization will be studied in response to specific processing tasks in Alzheimer's patients and in controls. It seems likely that these techniques will increase our understanding of the earlier and more fundamental changes which accompany the dementia process.

Another technology which is being applied to diagnosis of brain failure consists of various advanced techniques for the assessment of the brain's electrical activity. The traditional measure of the brain's

---

* One qualification is that whereas glucose is the major source of energy for the brain under most circumstances, alternative energy sources, such as those derived from the utilization of the so-called "ketone bodies," are also available to the brain.[13]

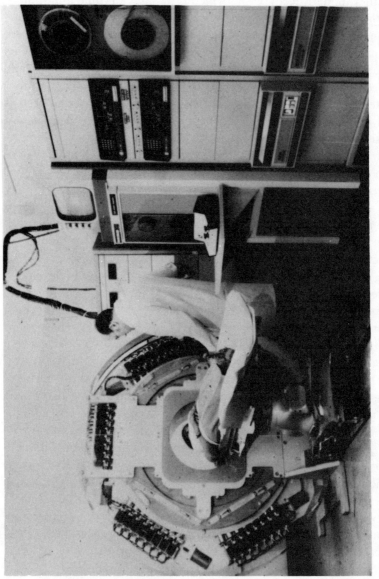

Figure 9.4. Position Emission Tomography. *Photograph coutesy of A. P. Wolf, Brookhaven National Laboratories, Associated Universities, Inc., Upton, N. Y. The PETT III apparatus shown above came from Dr. M. Ter-Pogossian, Washington University School of Medicine.*

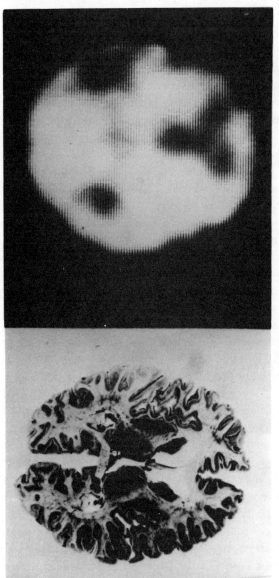

Figure 9.5 A Positron Emission Tomographic (PET) Scan of the Brain. Dark and light areas represent relative extent of glucose utilization by the living brain. *Photograph courtesy of S. H. Ferris, B. Reisberg, T. Farkas, A. P. Wolf, A. Alavi, D. Christman, J. Fowler, R. MacGregor, A. Goldman, R. Brill, and associates.*

electrical activity is the well-known electroencephalogram, or EEG. Since the development of the EEG by the psychiatrist Hans Berger approximately half a century ago, it has been widely applied, particularly to the diagnosis of neurological conditions such as epilepsy and space-occupying brain lesions such as tumors. The traditional EEG is read by a clinician, who looks for obvious abnormalities in the tracing. By identifying abnormal "spike activity," the clinician can diagnose an "epileptic focus," or by identifying an abnormal extent of slow activity over a particular brain area, the clinician may suspect the presence of an abnormal brain mass. Using traditional techniques, very little more information of diagnostic significance is available to the clinician reading a conventional EEG.

For several years researchers have utilized computers to analyze traditional EEGs in greater detail. This procedure, sometimes referred to as "quantitative EEG" or "QEEG," utilizes a computer to analyze the wave patterns.[14] These patterns are divided into several bands according to frequency, and the amount of activity in each band over a predetermined time period, such as an hour, is plotted. The resulting percentages provide a measure of the time devoted to each wave band in the EEG tracing.

In general, the more alert and/or anxious we are, the greater the percentage of fast wave activity on the EEG. When we relax, slower activity tends to predominate on the EEG. During sleep, except when we are dreaming, the EEG activity becomes even slower. A coma or a barbiturate overdose may produce still further slowing of the brain's electrical activity.

What happens to the brain's electrical activity in persons with Alzheimer's disease?

Since Alzheimer's involves the destruction of neurons in the outer layers of certain parts of the brain and a general slowing of thinking processes, we might expect a general slowing of the EEG wave bands to occur. This is precisely what is found.[15] Indeed, the relatively slow bands are especially notable over the temporal portion of the brain—the area where the Alzheimer's pathology predominates. Since the EEG is primarily a measure of the surface electrical activity coming from the outermost layers of the brain, it is particularly sensitive to a condition which affects the cortex, such as Alzheimer's disease.

Can the QEEG be utilized for the diagnosis of Alzheimer's disease?

At the present time, the EEG pattern in Alzheimer's disease is described as "characteristic, but not pathognomonic." This means that whereas certain predictable changes occur in the EEG pattern as the illness progresses, these changes are not unique. Hence the EEG changes identified thus far in Alzheimer's disease are not, by themselves, diagnostic of the condition. They are, currently, useful in confirming a diagnosis,[16,17,18,19] as well as in following the evolution of the condition.[20]

Multi-infarct dementia may produce changes on the EEG analogous to those which occur invariably in advanced Alzheimer's disease. If an M.I.D. patient has a particularly large hemorrhagic area close to the surface of the brain, then a general slowing in the EEG pattern will be found in the areas above the mass. In Alzheimer's the slowing would ordinarily tend to be diffuse and symmetrical, whereas in M.I.D. patients the slowing will most probably be unevenly distributed over the surface of the brain.[15]

One question which will almost certainly be clarified in the next decade is to what extent the early course of Alzheimer's disease is accompanied by concomitant changes in the brain's electrical activity. Also, relatively characteristic QEEG spectral patterns may be further identified.

Another area of investigation with respect to the brain's electrical activity is so-called "evoked potentials." These are patterns of electrical activity which are produced by the brain in the first fraction of a second after a sensory stimulus, such as a sound or a flash of light (see Figures 9–6 and 9–7). These evoked potential (EP) patterns can be recorded. Very elaborate computer techniques developed over the past decade enable the evoked potential patterns to be averaged and to be analyzed in great detail. These computer techniques are sometimes referred to as "neurometrics."[21]

Neurometric investigations have revealed that conditions which affect the brain often produce different EP electrical patterns. For example, it appears that conditions such as brain tumors can be diagnosed with considerable accuracy using neurometric techniques. More surprisingly, these techniques have been said to be useful in distinguishing children with learning disabilities from normal children. There is some preliminary evidence that EP patterns may be different in Alzheimer's patients.[21,22,23] Also, EP analyses are likely to be capable of revealing the presence of multiple, small infarcted areas.[24] It is quite possible that EP investigations currently underway will reveal patterns which are

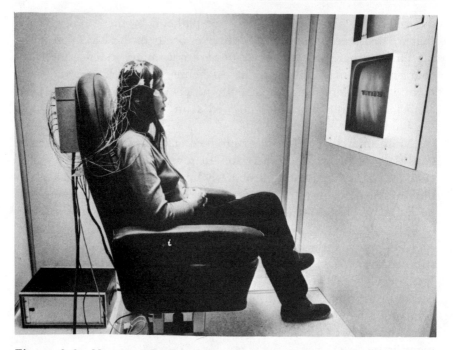

Figure 9.6 Neurometric Recording Apparatus. *Source:* The New York Times, *"Science Times,"* Tuesday, Mar. 11, 1980. Fred R. Conrad/NYT Pictures. © 1980 by The New York Times Company. Reprinted by permission.

diagnostically useful in senile dementia. If so, EP analysis might be an efficient, safe and relatively inexpensive means of confirming the clinician's diagnosis of the condition. EPs may prove to have additional diagnostic accuracy in determining the extent of involvement of deeper brain structures, and hence may aid in the differential diagnosis of Huntington's disease and of Parkinsonism or senile dementia with Parkinsonism.

The course and prognosis of senile dementia, and particularly of S.D.A.T., is one of the most important questions for the next decade. In particular, there is a great need to determine the evolution, course, prognosis, and natural history of early, very mild to moderately severe age-associated cognitive decline.

Each of the technologies discussed earlier is likely to prove of value in assisting scientists and, ultimately, clinicians in predicting the course and prognosis of senility. For example, it is possible that per-

At the University of California at San Diego, scientists use a computer to filter out electrical "noise" in the brain and isolate voltage changes relating to specific thoughts. In the experiment above, the sentence "It was his first day at work" is presented at the rate of one word every second. It results in a normal wave. But a nonsense sentence presented at the same rate produces a wave spike. At the N.Y.U. Medical Center, brain waves are studied in a special chamber [left] shielded against sound that might distract a subject and radiation that might interfere with brain wave recordings. Test material is flashed on the screen while the woman's brain waves are monitored from electrodes pasted to her scalp. An easy chair helps her relax to diminish noise associated with muscle movements.

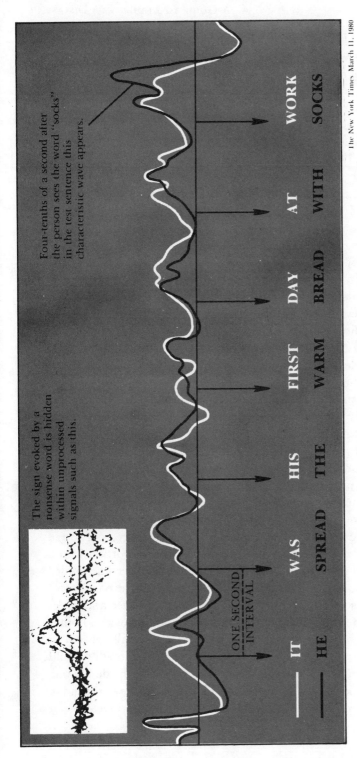

The sign evoked by a nonsense word is hidden within unprocessed signals such as this.

Four-tenths of a second after the person sees the word "socks" in the test sentence this characteristic wave appears.

ONE SECOND INTERVAL

IT   WAS   SPREAD HIS   THE   FIRST DAY   WARM   AT   WITH   WORK

HE   BREAD   SOCKS

The New York Times March 11, 1980

Figure 9.7 Evoked Potential Electrical Recordings in Response to Visual Word Stimuli. *Source:* The New York Times, "*Science Times,*" *Tuesday, Mar. 11, 1980.* © *1980 by The New York Times Company. Reprinted by permission.*

sons with overt evidence of atrophy as visualized on computerized tomographic scans will have a poorer prognosis than persons ostensibly with the same degree of impairment but without gross evidence of brain decay. Also, the area in which brain decay is located may be of prognostic significance.

The research establishments in the United States, and perhaps elsewhere, are already aware of the need to learn more about the prognosis and "natural history" of senile dementia. In 1979 the National Institute on Aging issued an announcement of its intent to award a contract to an institution capable of further defining the "natural history of senile dementia in a noninstitutional population."[25] Undoubtedly, future studies will answer many of the prognostic questions in the next decade. These answers should provide indirect benefits in the development of effective treatments for the dementias of late life. Since senile dementia is a chronic disorder, a truly significant treatment approach must ameliorate the condition over a period of years. For such a treatment to be properly assessed, it is obvious that the true course of the condition must be known.

The most important future investigations will continue to be those which bring us closer to an understanding of the causes of senile dementia and to the treatment and prevention of the condition. Exotic new technologies and techniques, once again, should assist in progress in these areas over the next decade. For example, researchers at the NIMH have developed a technique known as "brain transplant." It is possible to cut out portions of brain from one species of animal and to inject clumps of brain cells into the "ventricular," fluid-filled brain cavity of another animal, of a different species, and for the injected cells to grow and produce neuronal hormonal substances![26] This development may have enormous significance in aiding our investigations of the origins of senile dementia. For example, if one removes a portion of a dog brain containing senile plaques and injects that portion into a monkey brain, will the plaque spread? Will the monkey become senile? Even more significantly, it should be possible to remove portions of brain from persons who have died with Alzheimer's disease and inject clumps of cells containing plaques and tangles into monkeys and other animals. Assuming the clumps grow, will the PHFs, usually absent in monkey brains, survive? Will the plaques and tangles spread? Would antiviral agents, such as interferon, inhibit the spread of the dementia?

The number and variety of questions for which this new technique may eventually help provide answers are impressive and clearly not limited to those just outlined. However, in the absence of the necessary seminal investigations, further speculation would be premature.

Another, somewhat less exotic technique which is quite likely to tell us more about the origins of senile dementia is the scanning electron microscope (SEM). Very recent investigations, for example, utilizing this updated variant of electron microscopy have resulted in some quite interesting findings which would add directly to our earlier speculations regarding the origins of senile dementia. It has been shown that increased aluminum concentrations are found in the same brain cells as contain neurofibrillary tangles. Adjacent neurons, which do not contain PHFs, have lower aluminum concentrations in their nuclei.[27] This finding will undoubtedly lead scientists to reconsider the role of aluminum in Alzheimer's disease. The same technique, as well as future imaging and staining ultramicroscopic technologies, may implicate other substances which may lead us to a clearer understanding of the origins of brain failure.

We have already discussed in some detail new pharmacological agents which may lead us to an effective treatment approach to brain failure. Studies of prevention and of combinations of pharmacological agents may also prove fruitful. If viral agents play a role in the origins of S.D.A.T., then new antiviral agents, such as amantadine and interferon, may retard or even halt the condition. Interferon is a "species specific" substance which animals produce naturally, which appears to be effective in combating viral agents in general. In a certain sense, interferon may be to viruses what antibiotics are to bacteria—a generally effective treatment approach. Using recombinant genetic "gene splicing" techniques, scientists have reportedly succeeded in producing human interferon in laboratory bacteria.[28] This breakthrough may enable scientists to produce sufficient quantities of this very rare material substance for it to be a commercially practical antiviral treatment.[29,30] Sufficient quantities will probably become available for an investigation of the substance in the treatment of Alzheimer's disease.

An exciting new model may further aid in the investigation and development of effective treatments for Alzheimer's disease. As mentioned in Chapter 3, scientists in Canada have succeeded in "transferring" human PHFs to cellular tissue cultures. Specifically, it is possible to grow fetal neuronal cells in tissue culture. If one adds a homogenate composed of crushed brain material from Alzheimer's-affected brains to the tissue culture medium, some of the cultured cells develop classical PHFs! Furthermore, the Alzheimer's homogenate can be diluted up to 100,000 times without losing its ability to produce PHFs in the cell culture medium.[31]

The tissue culture model must be further refined before it will be useful as a "bioassay" for the testing of possible treatments of S.D.A.T. Human fetal brain material is difficult to obtain. Umberto de Boni, the scientist who has been primarily responsible for the development of the technique, must go to a local obstetric ward and wait for an abortion. He quickly removes the fetus to his laboratory and cultures the brain material. Equally laborious is searching for PHFs once the brain homogenate has been added. Since the PHFs grow only very sparsely, a technician must search the culture medium before he feels confident in concluding that no PHFs are present. Fetal neuronal cells do not divide and are not readily available, hence the entire laborious process must be repeated for each experiment.

In the next decade, these tissue culture models of Alzheimer's disease may be developed and refined so that they become a more easily available qualitative and perhaps even quantitative model of the illness. They might then provide a medium for the rapid testing of pharmacological agents for efficacy in the treatment of S.D.A.T.

The time savings over the laborious long-term clinical trials which are now required to test new treatments may be decisive in enabling scientists to develop a cure for senile dementia before the next century. Considering the significant advances which have been described in this book, virtually all of which have been made in the past 25 years, such optimism may be justifiable.

Notes

1. Thaler, H. T., Ferber, P. W., and Rottenberg, D. A., A statistical method for determining the proportions of gray matter, white matter, and CSF using computed tomography. *Neuroradiology* 16: 133–135, 1978.
2. Roberts, M. A., Caird, F. I., Grossart, K. W., and Steven, J. L., Computerized tomography in the diagnosis of cerebral atrophy. *J. Neurol. Neurosurg. Psychiat.* 39: 905–915, 1976.
3. Claveria, L. E., Moseley, I. F., and Stevenson, J. F., The clinical significance of "cerebral atrophy" as shown by C.A.T. In G. H. du Boulay and I. F. Moseley (eds.), *The First European Seminar on Computerized Axial Tomography in Clinical Practice,* Springer-Verlag, Berlin, 1977, pp. 213–217.
4. Gado, M., Hughes, C., Naidich, T., and Moran, C., Atrophy versus ag-

ing, Symposium on C.T., Las Vegas, April 1979, Abstract. In *J. Comput. Assist. Tomogr.* 3: 563, 1979.

5. Huckman, M. S., Fox, J., and Topel, J., The validity of criteria for the evaluation of cerebral atrophy by computed tomography. *Radiology* 116: 85–92, 1975.

6. Du Boulay, G., Fairbairn, D., and Paden, R. S., Precise re-positioning of the head for serial CT examinations. Neuroradiology 16: 625–626, 1978.

7. De Leon, M. J., Ferris, S. H., George, A. E., Reisberg, B., Kricheff, I. I., and Gershon, S., Computed tomography evaluations of brain-behavior relationships in senile dementia of the Alzheimer's type. *Neurobiology of Aging: Experimental and Clinical Research,* Vol. 1, No. 1, 69–79, 1980.

8. George, A. E., de Leon, M. J., Ferris, S. H., and Kricheff, I. I., Parenchymal CT correlates of senile dementia: Loss of gray-white matter discriminability. American Society of Neuroradiology, 18th Annual Meeting, Los Angeles, Calif., Mar. 16–21, 1980.

9. Brinkman, S. D., Sarwar, M., and Levin, H. S., Quantified computerized tomographic (CT) changes in normal aging and dementia: Relationship to behavior. Paper presented at the Gerontological Society 31st Annual Meeting, Dallas, Nov. 16–20, 1978.

10. Hachinski, V. C., Iliff, L. D., Zilhka, E., du Boulay, G. H., McAllister, V. L., Marshall, J., Ross Russell, R. W., and Symon, L., Cerebral blood flow in dementia. *Arch. Neurol.* 32: 632–637, 1975.

11. Ingvar, D. H., Brun, A., Hagberg, B., and Gustafson, L., Regional cerebral blood flow in the dominant hemisphere in confirmed cases of Alzheimer's disease, Pick's disease, and multi-infarct dementia: Relationship to clinical symptomatology and neuropathological findings. In *Alzheimer's Disease: Senile Dementia and Related Disorders (Aging,* Vol. 7), ed. by R. Katzman, R. D. Terry, and K. L. Bick, Raven Press, New York, 1978.

12. Yamaguchi, F., Meyer, J. S., Yamamoto, M., Sakai, F., and Shaw, T., Noninvasive cerebral blood flow measurements in dementia. *Arch Neurol.,* 37: 410–418, 1980.

13. Hawkins, R. A., and Biebuyck, J. F., Ketone bodies are selectively used by individual brain regions. *Science* 205: 325–327, 1979.

14. Itil, T. M., Quantitative pharmaco-electroencephalography: Use of computerized cerebral biopotentials in psychotropic drug research. In *Modern Problems of Pharmacopsychiatry,* Vol. 8, *Psychotropic Drugs and the Human EEG,* volume ed. Turan M. Itil, series eds. Th. A. Ban, F. A. Freyhan, P. Pinchot, and W. Pöldinger, S. Karger, Basel, 1974, pp. 43–75.

15. Müller, H. F., and Schwartz, G., Electroencephalograms and autopsy findings in geropsychiatry. *J. Geront.* 33: 504–513, 1978.

16. Green, M. A., Stevenson, L. D., Fonseen, J. E., and Wortis, S. B., Cerebral biopsy in patients with presenile dementia. *Dis. Nerv. Syst.* 13: 303–307, 1952.
17. Letemendia, F., and Pampiglione, G., Clinical and electroencephalographic observations in Alzheimer's disease. *J. Neurol. Neurosurg. Psychiat.* 21: 167–172, 1958.
18. Swain, J. M., Electroencephalographic abnormalities in presenile atrophy. *Neurology* 9: 722–727, 1959.
19. Gordon, E. B., and Sim, M., The EEG in presenile dementia. *J. Neurol. Neurosurg. Psychiat.* 30: 285–291, 1967.
20. Johannesson, G., Brun, A., Gustafson, I., and Ingvar, D. H., EEG in presenile dementia related to cerebral blood flow and autopsy findings. *Acta Neurol. Scand.* 56: 89–103, 1977.
21. John, E. R., Karmel, B. Z., Corning, W. C., Easton, P., Brown, D., Ahn, H., John, M., Harmony, T., Prichep, L., Toro, A., Gerson, I., Bartlett, F., Thatcher, R., Kaye, H., Valdes, P., and Schwartz, E., Neurometrics. *Science* 196: 1393–1410, 1977.
22. John, E. R., *Functional Neuroscience,* Vol. II, *Neurometrics: Clinical Applications of Quantitative Electrophysiology,* Erlbaum Associates, New York, 1977.
23. Straumanis, J. J., Shagass, C., and Schwartz, M., Visually evoked cerebral response changes associated with chronic brain syndromes and aging. *J. Geront.* 20: 498–506, 1965.
24. Tsamoto, T., Hirose, N., Nonaka, S., and Takahashi, M., Cerebrovascular disease: Changes in somatosensory evoked potentials associated with unilateral lesions. *Electroencephalography and Clin. Neurophysiol.* 35: 463–473, 1973.
25. Sources Sought Announcement, No. NIH-AG-80-10, Dec. 13, 1979, "Senile Dementia: Natural History in a Noninstitutionalized Population," NIH Guide for Grants and Contracts, Supplement, U.S. Department of Health, Education, and Welfare.
26. Perlow, M. J., Freed, W. J., Seiger, A., Olson, L., and Wyatt, R. J., Brain grafts reduce motor abnormalities produced by destruction of nigrostriatal dopamine system. *Science* 204: 643–647, 1979.
27. Liss, L., Ebner, K., Couri, D., and Long, J., Correlation of aluminum content with morphological changes and predisposing factors. Presented at the Gerontological Society, 32nd Annual Scientific Meeting, Washington, D.C., Nov. 25–29, 1979.
28. Taniguichi, T., Sakai, M., Fujii-Kuriyama, Y., Maramatsu, M., Kobayashi, S., and Sudo, T., Construction and identification of a bacterial plasmid containing the human fibroblast interferon gene sequence. *Proc. Jap. Acad.* 55B: 461–469, 1979.
29. New York Times News Service, Scientists create a virus fighter. *San Jose Mercury,* Jan. 17, 1980.

30. Bishop, J., Proving medical value of interferon may take a long time. *Wall Street Journal,* Feb. 5, 1980.
31. Crapper, D. R., and De Boni, U., Etiological factors in dementia. International Society for Neurochemistry Satellite Meeting on Aging of the Brain and Dementia, Florence, Italy, Aug. 27–29, 1979, Abstracts.

Selected Annotated Bibliography

I. Edited texts on senile dementia and Alzheimer's disease

1. *Aging and Dementia*, ed. by W. Lynn Smith and Marcel Kinsbourne, SP Books Division of Spectrum Publications, Inc., New York, 1977, 244 pages. Probably the best edited introductory text in the field. Ideal for medical students and other health professionals with no technical knowledge of the area.
2. *The Aging Brain and Senile Dementia*, ed. by Kalidas Nandy and Ira Sherwin, Plenum Press, New York, 1977, 307 pages. A good intermediate edited text which emphasizes pathological and physiological changes accompanying senile dementia.
3. *Aging*, Vol. 2, *Genesis and Treatment of Psychologic Disorders in the Elderly*, ed. by S. Gershon and A. Raskin, Raven Press, New York, 1975, 277 pages. Contains several review chapters on pharmacological treatments of senile dementia. Also contains some basic chapters on cognitive assessment, physiology, and pathology.
4. *Aging*, Vol. 7, *Alzheimer's Disease: Senile Dementia and Related Disorders*, ed. by Robert Katzman, Robert D. Terry, and Katherine L. Bick, Raven Press, New York, 1978, 595 pages. The most comprehensive and definitive collection of work in the area of senile dementia which is available at this time.

II. Comprehensive overviews of senile dementia and Alzheimer's disease

1. TORACK, R. M., *The Pathologic Physiology of Dementia, with Indications for Diagnosis and Treatment,* Springer-Verlag, Berlin, 1978, 155 pages. Perhaps the only book-length single-authored work on the subject currently available. This treatise is of variable quality. Although the work is probably too obtuse for the novitiate, specialists in the field will find some of the theories proposed intriguing. The author's comprehensive approach to this formidable undertaking is to be commended, and the result is provocative and stimulating for other experts in the field.
2. FISK, A. A., Senile dementia, Alzheimer-type (SDAT): A review of present knowledge. *Wisconsin Med. J.* 78: 29–33, 1979. A brief overview which could serve as an introduction for physicians and other professionals.
3. "Information on Alzheimer's Disease." Pamphlet available from the National Institute on Aging, National Institute of Health, Bethesda, Md. 20014. An introduction which is of considerable value to laymen.

III. Etiology of senescent brain failure

1. TOMLINSON, B. E., BLESSED, G., and ROTH, M., Observations on the brains of non-demented old people. *J. Neurol. Sci.* 7: 331–356, 1968. A classic article which will become an important historical document.
2. TOMLINSON, B. E., BLESSED, G., and ROTH, M., Observations on the brains of demented old people. *J. Neurol. Sci.* 11: 205–242, 1970. A companion article to the 1968 article.
3. DeBONI, U., DALTON, A. J., SCHOLOTTERER, M. A., and CRAPPER, D. R., Senile dementia: Recent concepts of pathophysiology. *Research in Dementia: Proceedings of a Colloquium of the Ontario Psycho-Geriatric Association,* Research Bulletin 3: 1–15, 1977.
4. WISNIEWSKI, H. M., BRUCE, M. E. and FRASER, H., Infectious etiology of neurotic (senile) plaques in mice. *Science* 190: 1108–1110, 1975.
5. WISNIEWSKI, H. M., and SOIFER, D., Neurofibrillary pathology: Current status and research perspectives. *Mechanisms of Ageing and Development* 9: 119–142, 1979.
6. PERL, D. P., and BRODY, A. R., Alzheimer's disease: X-ray spectrometric evidence of aluminum accumulation in neurofibrillary tangle-bearing neurons. *Science* 208: 297–299, 1980.
7. HACHINSKI, V. C., LASSEN, N. A., and MARSHALL, J., Multi-infarct dementia: A cause of mental deterioration in the elderly. *Lancet,* 11: 207–221, 1974. A classic introduction to this important dementia etiology.

8. HESTON, L. L., and MASTRI, A. R., The genetics of Alzheimer's disease: Associations with hematologic malignancy and Down's syndrome. *Arch. Gen. Psychiat.* 34: 976–981, 1977.

9. COOK, R. H., WARD, B. E., and AUSTIN, J. H., Studies in aging of the brain: IV. Familial. Alzheimer disease; relation to transmissible dementia, aneuploidy and microtubular defects. *Neurology* 29: 1402–1412, 1979.

10. CRAPPER, D. R., QUITTKAT, S., and DE BONI, U., Altered chromatin confirmation in Alzheimer's disease. *Brain* 102: 483–495, 1979.

11. JARVIK, L. F., Memory loss and its possible relationship to chromosomal changes. In *Psychopharmacology and Aging*, ed. by EISDORFER, C. and W. E. FANN, Vol. 6 in *Advances in Behavioral Biology*, Plenum Press, New York, 1973, pp. 145–150.

12. WISNIEWSKI, K., HOWE, J., WILLIAMS, D. G., and WISNIEWSKI, H. M., Precocious aging and dementia in patients with Down's syndrome. *Biol. Psychiat.* 13: 619–627, 1978.

IV. Pharmacotherapy of senile dementia and age-associated cognitive decline

A. Edited texts

1. *Geriatric Psychopharmacology*, ed. by KALIDAS NANDY, Elsevier/North-Holland, New York, 1979. A comprehensive work with several good reviews of specific areas.
2. *CNS Aging and Its Neuropharmacology: Experimental and Clinical Aspects*, Vol. 15 of *Interdisciplinary Topics in Gerontology*, volume ed. W. MEIER-RUGE, series ed. H. P. VON HAHN, S. Karger, Basel, 218 pages. Contains several chapters which would be of value to investigators in the field.
3. *Physician's Handbook on Psychotherapeutic Drug Use in the Aged*, ed. by GENE D. COHEN and THOMAS CROOK, Mark Powley Associates, Inc., in press. When available, this slim, readable work will provide a valuable introduction to the area.

B. Comprehensive, chapter-length overviews

1. REISBERG, B., FERRIS, S. H., and GERSHON, S., Overview of drug treatment of cognitive decline. *Amer. J. Psychiat.*, in press. A comprehensive introduction to the area.
2. REISBERG, B., FERRIS, S. H., and GERSHON, S., Pharmacotherapy of senile dementia. In *Psychopathology in the Aged*, ed. by JONATHAN O. COLE and

JAMES E. BARRETT. Raven Press, New York, pp. 233-261. Provides a detailed review of the current status of drug treatment of the condition.

C. Selected important pharmacotherapeutic references

1. RASKIN, A., GERSHON, S., CROOK, T. H., SATHANANTHAN, G., and FERRIS, S., The effects of hyperbaric and normobaric oxygen on cognitive impairment in the elderly. *Arch. Gen. Psychiat.* 35: 50–56, 1978. A detailed report of the most important and most thorough scientific examination of the efficacy of this treatment modality conducted to date.
2. YESAVAGE, J. A., TINKLENBERG, J., HOLLISTER, L. E., and BERGER, P. A., Vasodilators in senile dementia: A review of the literature. *Arch. Gen. Psychiat.* 36: 220–223, 1979. An excellent, detailed review of these important pharmacotherapeutic agents.
3. JARVIK, L. F., and MILNE, J. F., Gerovital-H3: A review of the literature. In *Aging*, Vol. 2, ed. by S. GERSHON and A. RASKIN, Raven Press, New York, 1975, pp. 203–227. An important review of this controversial area.
4. *Nutrition and the Brain*, Vol. 5, *Choline and Lecithin in Brain Disorders*, ed. by A. BARBEAU, J. H. GROWDEN, and R. J. WURTMAN, Raven Press, New York, 1979, 456 pages. Contains several chapters describing the status of current efforts to improve cognition with neurotransmitter agonists and precursors.
5. FERRIS, S. H., REISBERG, B., and GERSHON, S., Neuropeptide modulation of cognition and memory in humans, Chap. 15 in *Aging in the 1980's*, ed. by L. W. POON, published by American Psychological Association, 1980, pp. 212–220. An up-to-date overview of this important new area.

V. Psychotherapy and psychotherapeutic interventions

1. FOLSOM, J. C., Reality orientation for the elderly mental patient. *J. Geriatric Psychiat.* 1: 291–307, 1968.
2. BRADNO, J., and SELTZER, J., Resocialization therapy through group processes with senile patients in a geriatric hospital. *Gerontologist* 8(3): 211–214, 1968.
3. BURNSIDE, IRENE M., Group therapy with regressed aged people. In I. M. BURNSIDE (ed.), *Nursing and the Aged*, McGraw-Hill, New York, 1976.
4. SILVER, A., Group psychotherapy with senile psychiatric patients. *Geriatrics* 5: 147–150, 1950.
5. BROWNE, H. E., and WINKELMAYER, R., A structured music therapy in geriatrics. In E. T. GASTON (ed.), *Music in Therapy*, Macmillan, New York, 1968.
6. PALMER, M. D., Music therapy in a comprehensive program of treatment

and rehabilitation for the geriatric resident. *J. Music Therapy* 14: 190–197, 1977.

VI. Aging and institutionalization

1. BUTLER, ROBERT N., *Why Survive? Being Old in America,* Harper & Row, New York, 1975, 496 pages. This overview of the sociopolitical, economic, and medical context of aging in the United States has won a Pulitzer Prize. It is a classic and invaluable work.
2. OTTEN, JANE, and SHELLEY, FLORENCE D., *When Your Parents Grow Old,* Funk & Wagnalls, a division of Thomas Y. Crowell Co., Inc., New York, 1976, 291 pages. Contains information which will probably prove of interest and value to laymen.
3. MANARD, BARBARA BOLLING, KART, CARRY STEVEN, and VAN GILS, DIRK W. L., *Old-Age Institutions,* D. C. Heath & Company, Lexington, Mass., 1975, 157 pages. Contains useful statistical and background information based upon surveys of institutional facilities for the aged.
4. MANARD, BARBARA BOLLING, WOEHLE, RALPH E., and JAMES M. HEILMAN, *Better Homes for the Old,* D. C. Heath & Company, Lexington, Mass., 1977, 152 pages. Contains a concrete and provocative analysis of ways to improve and assess the quality of homes for the aged.
5. BERGMANN, K., FOSTER, E. M., JUSTICE, A. W., and MATTHEWS, V., Management of the demented elderly patient in the community. *Brit. J. Psychiat.* 132: 441–449, May 1978.

VII. Assessment of cognitive decline and senile dementia

A. Psychological and psychiatric assessments

1. *Psychiatric Symptoms and Cognitive Loss in the Elderly: Evaluation and Assessment Techniques,* ed. by A. RASKIN and L. F. JARVIK, Halsted Press, John Wiley & Sons, Inc., New York, 1979, 308 pages. An important introduction to this area.

B. Technological advances in the assessment of cognitive decline

1. DE LEON, M. J., FERRIS, S. H., GEORGE, A. E., REISBERG, B., KRICHEFF, I. I., and GERSHON, S., Computed tomography evaluations of brain-behavior relationships in senile dementia of the Alzheimer's type. *Neurobiology of Aging: Experimental and Clinical Research,* Vol. 1, No. 1, 69–79, 1980. A technical introduction to the possibilities of assessment in this area utilizing sophisticated, innovative techniques.

2. LASSEN, N. A., INGVAR, D. H., and SKINHØJ, E., Brain function and blood flow. *Scientific American,* October 1978, pp. 62–71. A lucid explanation of cerebral blood flow methodology.

3. JOHN, E. R., KARMEL, B. Z., CORNING, W. C., EASTON, P., BROWN, D., AHN, H., JOHN, M., HARMONY, T., PRICHEP, L., TORO, A., GERSON, I., BARTLETT, F., THATCHER, R., KAYE, H., VALDES, P., and SCHWARTZ, E., Neurometrics. *Science* 196: 1393–1410, 1977. A classic description of these increasingly important, sophisticated, electrophysiological assessments.

4. MERSKEY, H., BALL, M. J., BLUME, W. T., FOX, A. J., Fox, H., HERSCH, E. L., KRAL, V. A., and PALMER, R. B., Relationships between psychological measurements and cerebral organic changes in Alzheimer's disease. *Journal Canadien des Sciences Neurologiques* 7: 45–49, 1980. Describes an interesting study of EEG/CT/psychometric interrelationships.

VIII. Journals and periodicals

1. *Geriatrics*
   Published monthly by Harcourt Brace Jovanovich Health Care Publications, 757 Third Avenue, New York, N.Y. 10017. This journal for the primary-care physician contains occasional review articles of interest to professionals working with patients having Alzheimer's disease or senile dementia.

2. *The Gerontologist*
   Published bimonthly by the Gerontological Society, 1835 K Street, N.W., Washington, D.C. 20006. Contains original articles on the sociology of aging.

3. *Journal of Gerontology*
   Published bimonthly by the Gerontological Society, 1835 K Street, N.W., Washington, D.C. 20006. The official organ of the Gerontological Society, devoted to research on aging, this contains many important original contributions to the field.

4. *Journal of the American Geriatrics Society*
   Published monthly by the American Geriatrics Society Inc., 10 Columbus Circle, New York, N.Y. 10019. The official organ of the American Geriatrics Society, a medical organization, this journal contains original articles of particular interest to physicians.

5. *Age and Aging*
   Published quarterly by Bailliere Tindall, 35 Red Lion Square, London WCIR 4SG. The official journal of the British Geriatrics Society and of the British Society for Research on Aging. Contains many excellent original articles of interest to investigators.

Index